Standing in Two Places:

A New Landscape of Motherhood

Ashley Dyson

D1293916

Aberdeen Bay

Atlanta - Beijing - Harbin - Washington, D.C.

Aberdeen Bay
Published by Aberdeen Bay, an imprint of Champion Writers.
www.aberdeenbay.com

Copyright © Ashley Dyson, 2009

All rights reserved. No part of this publication may be reproduced, stored in a database or retrieval system, or transmitted, in any form or by any means, without the prior written permission of the publisher. For information on obtaining permission for use of material from this publication, please visit the publisher's website at www.aberdeenbay.com.

Grateful acknowledgment is made for permission to quote from *On Fertile Ground: A Natural History of Human Reproduction* by Peter T. Ellison, pp.7-8, Cambridge, Mass.: Harvard University Press, copyright © 2001 by the President and Fellows of Harvard College.

PUBLISHER'S NOTE

Aberdeen Bay is not responsible for the accuracy of this book—including but not limited to events, people, dates, and locations.

International Standard Book Number
ISBN-13: 978-1-60830-014-3
ISBN-10: 1-60830-014-5

Printed in the United States of America.

Author Bio

Ashley Dyson graduated from Middlebury College and received an MFA in Creative Writing from George Mason University. She lives in New York with her husband and two children.

For Patrick Dyson, of course

Author's Note

I did not change the locations or the names of agencies or buildings in this book, but I have changed all of the names of the people who played such important roles in it. My reason for making these changes was to protect and honor their privacy.

All author royalties will be donated to The Center for Surrogate Parenting.

Standing in Two Places:

A New Landscape of Motherhood

"For, indeed, in the social jungle of human existence there is no feeling of being alive without a sense of identity."

— Erik H. Erikson, *Identity: Youth and Crisis*

Prologue

Lately memoirs have disappointed me. So I have been reading biographies, historical biographies especially, for their objectivity in telling a good story about an interesting life. But I am drawn to the memoir for what the biography lacks, and that is the constant voice of its subject, piecing together a life that is still in the process of living. In the last few years memoirs have put me off, at least many of the contemporary ones (not Joan Didion's) where every page seems to be a contest in suffering that hovers close to shock-value; a bit like reality TV. I find that when I finish reading one of these memoirs I haven't learned anything new. Yes, the resilience of the human spirit is once again confirmed, but I already knew that. A human being surviving heroin binges, prison, abuse in all forms, botched surgeries, and cruel parents (whether fabricated or not) is fascinating, but it seems to me that in these memoirs more emphasis is placed on the just-getting-by side of living, the defensive side, as opposed to the living part, the living well part, the living peacefully part despite all the drama, and how exactly one achieves that.

Perhaps what I seek is a good reason, a greater purpose, a justification for unveiling one's secrets, one's suffering, one's family dramas. I grew up in a family of proud and private southerners; when I asked my grandmother how she got over her grief after my grandfather died suddenly at the breakfast table one morning, just weeks before they were to begin retirement together and travel the world, she replied, "I took care of my roses. Then I confirmed my trip on the Queen Elizabeth II around the world. I got moving, that's what I did. That's just what you do." I remember sitting next to her on the couch and how, as she spoke, her entire body language changed: her back straightened, she pushed her shoulders back, she raised her chin and peered down at me as if my question had been foolish. I suddenly felt small, and my petite, 100-pound grandmother seemed like a giant to me.

And years later when she lay dying in the very bed in which she was born, she didn't want to talk about dying or the pain, or the bitch of watching her body waste away, she wanted to talk about life. She wanted my mother and father and my brother and me to sit down next to her bed and just talk; she still wanted to laugh, she still wanted a glass of Chivas Regal at six o'clock (even if it sat untouched on the bedside table). What she didn't want was drama: no grief-stricken visitors, no sympathy phone calls, no bed-side vigils. We screened all cards and flowers that alluded to death or sickness. Her companion, a retired doctor living down in Jacksonville, Florida had no idea that she was sick, and that's how she wanted it because dying was private. Like sex, money, and body weight, there were things in life that should remain private. For my grandmother, and for the rest of us who continued to live after she was gone, living a dignified life and a private life were one in the same; never did you hang your white wash out to dry.

Drama happens, as does pain and suffering and all of the ingredients in those page-turning memoirs, there is no doubt about that, and it finds its way into every life, whether invited in or not. I have spent a large portion of my life enacting every possible strategy to control it, deny it, diffuse it, and run from it, and wouldn't you know it, on the night of September 24, 2002, I found myself in the middle of one of the oldest dramas in the history of women: surviving childbirth or dying from it.

It was clear from my first realization of motherhood that, for me, this rite of passage, believed so innately central to a woman's life, was not following the script. Mine was nothing like the childbirths I had witnessed, where a party of friends and family gathered in the birthing room immediately after the baby's birth to celebrate with cigars and champagne. Minutes after my daughter's birth, I began to hemorrhage. Blood transfusions, and what I like to think was sheer will by both my doctor and myself, brought me back. I was then sequestered in intensive care, visitors were turned away, phone calls were not returned. Days later I was moved back into a regular hospital room and finally able to hold my daughter for the first time. I remember I lay in bed with my daughter in my arms, listening to the frantic ring of the telephone, not yet conscious that my quiet war with drama had begun. The telephone rang incessantly throughout the day, at odd hours of the night; worried, impatient, sometimes angry voices filled the voicemail with questions: *What exactly happened? Is Ashley going to live? Is something wrong with the baby? Have you even had the baby? I guess I will hear from you when I hear from you —* then a dial tone. After that I unplugged the phone and spent four more weeks in the hospital, then two glorious years hiding in the cocoon of new motherhood, distancing myself from that night and its consequences, though somehow I knew it would all re-emerge when the question of more children inevitably surfaced, as it did.

What followed next was a world I had never imagined, the world of surrogacy, a controversial practice in its own right (*Baby M*, talk about drama). I entered a surrogacy arrangement with my eyes open, but with my head turned away, for I sensed in every corner, in every shadow, in every step along the way, that drama lingered. So I coasted. I had been coasting along for the past three years, comfortable with myself and with my decision to use the help of a surrogate. I coasted through the headache of all the legal work, through the stress of finding a clinic in a state where surrogacy is legal, since in our home state of New York it is not; I coasted through the months of waiting for the agency to match us with a surrogate, in the phone call and actual meeting of our surrogate, Norah; I coasted through IVF, through the drugs and procedures, and calmly watched as the doctor inserted our embryos into Norah's uterus; and it is here, for only a few seconds, that my coasting came to an abrupt stop. Watching on the screen as the catheter penetrated the cervix and the actual release of two embryos could be seen, I remember feeling a second of nothingness. Standing in that small room I felt myself inch closer to the door, partly to respect Norah's privacy and partly because I felt my role had begun to diminish: who was I supposed to be now? Was I like the sports fan, cheering my embryos and Norah on? Or was I more like a supportive friend, wishing all present the best of luck before I went on my merry way? Or was I simply a witness to this miraculous procedure in artificial reproductive technology, a number to add to the statistics?

Norah's role was obvious, it loomed large and important as I held her arm and escorted her out of the room; but for me, the exact definition of my role was unclear.

Motherhood is a high stakes world, even in the most ideal and normal of circumstances. There are rites of passage a woman must go through to earn the title of mother: love, in some form, conception, the body growing larger, baby showers, strangers and friends oohing and ahhing over a pregnant belly, and finally the labor of childbirth. Funerals and marriage, childbirth and baptisms, debutante balls and bar mitzvahs, human beings need their rituals, as both an inner validation, as well as a public one. Human rituals are ingrained in our civilization for a reason, not because they necessarily give us the answers on how to survive life's transitions, but because they give us a framework for our new roles—be it mother, father, widow or widower. Rituals give us an official place to begin, and that is something. But for a woman whose fetus grows inside another, what rite of passage is there for her? What rituals are there to define her role? With my daughter it was a long, physical labor, testing my strength and will, reaffirming the tenacity I had always suspected intrinsically in women; but with my second child, I was more like the man, the father who, for nine months, goes about his business as usual, waiting for the healthy baby to be delivered, all clean and fresh and blanketed, into his arms. Surely my secret desire during the nine months of Norah's pregnancy to hide, to escape—not metaphorically, but literally to jump ship, skip town, flee, was something perhaps more biological than egocentric.

Of course I did not run away, not in body at least, but in mind I began to retreat, as I slowly realized that I was in conflict with myself. I was a mother to a three-year-old and a mother-to-be to a baby growing inside the womb of another woman living four states away; I had willingly, enthusiastically, signed up for surrogacy then discovered, a bit too late, that perhaps I didn't have the right stuff for this arrangement; there was my old self, delighting in the anticipation of another baby, grateful for the good fortune of finding Norah, and there was a new self emerging, full of shame and anxiety over the fact that I would not be carrying the baby, and a strong desire to crawl in a hole and hide. If ever there was a time in my life when I needed to stand tall and proceed with a deep sense of self, this was it; but the person whom I had believed myself to be, the designated driver, the independent problem-solver, the disciple of a grandmother who had always pulled up her boot straps: *you get moving, that's what I did, that's just what you do,* that person had disappeared under the weight of this crisis. And that's what it was, a crisis, an "identity crisis," a phrase I borrowed from the psychologist, Erik H. Erikson, and clung to like a talisman during the nine months of Norah's pregnancy, and even to this day. Though Erikson had coined the phrase to refer to a turning point in an adolescent's development, his book, my bible, *Identity: Youth and Crisis,* became for me, a thirty-five-year-old woman, a place to begin in my search for identity.

Surrogacy is just one of the many reproductive technologies that is changing the way we view parenthood and childbirth, it is transforming the most basic of human biological relationships: that of parent and child. My generation and our children are the subjects of this reproductive revolution, and much of this terrain, it seems, must be figured out on a trial and error basis; to be sure, there is much drama to be found here. But there is also a great responsibility to push through the muck of drama in order to ascend with the understanding of what Erikson calls, "The Life Cycle, the Epigenesis of Identity," in which growth, over a human being's lifespan, is defined by "conflicts, inner and outer, which the vital personality weathers, re-emerging from each crisis with an increased sense of inner unity, with an increase of good judgment, and an increase in the capacity 'to do well' according to his own standards and to the standards of those who are significant to him." In essence it is the discovery, or better, a reminder, that we have the capability to be reborn again and again; we can adapt, and live well.

I wrote this book in the heat of battle against myself and

my notions of motherhood and growing up. Surrogacy was the back-drop to a larger theme: love. Love, as defined by fluidity, growth, change, all of those terrifying and elusive ingredients in the business of growing up. If not for love, what other reason is there to willingly throw oneself headlong into the unknown? For what I finally discovered as I stumbled, fell, and hid through the nine months of Norah's pregnancy, was the necessity of the falling, of the cowardice, of the retreat, and the subsequent getting up, facing up, and opening the door, if I was to truly own, and own up to, my new role. It is the stagnancy of life that one should fear most, the standing on the elevator and never going anywhere, the immature love whose passions never evolve beyond sloppy kissing, the embryo that never grows larger than the pit of a peach, or the girl that turns away from the truth that what has been lost has been replaced with possibility. The possibility of something wonderful, something new and uncharted, that draws her out of her room ready to begin again.

It is for my husband, my two daughters, and dear Norah, that I wrote this book. In stark contrast to me, they proved unwavering in their roles. For everything which I kept hidden and lost, they uncovered and replenished with love, resolve, and truth.

September 23, 2005

My daughter turns three tomorrow, my nine-week-old embryo is in Indiana, my husband is in L.A. on business, and I am in bed in New York flipping through a book entitled, *Homemade Baby Food*; it is a Friday night. I have not looked at this book in over a year, and as I turn the pages I realize that I have highlighted, a lot. Thick strips of glowing, yellow marker highlight paragraphs and sentences throughout the book — when did I do this? I cannot remember. I stop at a heavily highlighted page and read:

> You may be tempted to open a can of applesauce or canned vegetables and mash them up thinking you have made 'fresh' food. This defeats the purpose of making baby food. Canned foods or canned fruits have additives, particularly sodium and/or sugar, which baby doesn't need.

Along with recipes for Pureed Chicken Liver and Hint of Mint Soup, I am warned against biological, chemical and physical hazards; nitrates, botulism, choking; hot spots and burns; clean versus sanitary; bacteria versus microorganisms; refrigerator temperatures, clean hands, and the nutritional benefits of steaming. There is a chapter on allergies and a brief lesson on the history of the word 'allergy' (it's Greek). I flip to the back of the book, searching for a dessert section. There is a recipe for a first birthday cake, and one last reminder: "The first birthday is the most special, so put some time into the cake."
And I highlighted all of it.
Soon after my daughter's birth, when my doctor told me

that I could not carry another baby, I was oddly fine with it. After seven weeks in the hospital, a few blood transfusions, two more weeks in the hospital's hotel, and countless MRIs to monitor a large part of my placenta that refused to come out, my daughter and I had survived her birth, and she was healthy. Plus, I had the added comfort of choices: there were other ways to have more children. For the first year of my daughter's life I was safe from the question I came to fear most: when are you having more kids? I didn't go out much that first year; I slept, scrubbed my hands with antibacterial soap, fell deeply in love with my daughter, and evidently did a lot of highlighting in books. It was sometime between my daughter's first and second birthdays, when she began to grow hair and teeth and to walk and talk and coo at anything with a face, that the question entered my life. I learned that the mere fact of having a child invites inquiries, advice, admonishments from perfect strangers, especially when you live in New York, a city not known for its reticence. On cold days strangers warned that my daughter's sweater was too thin, that she needed a hat; that pacifier-use guaranteed a future smoker; that candy will rot children's teeth out; and why hadn't I gotten my daughter's ears pierced, baby girls look so adorable with little pearl earrings! I grew up in Virginia, my mother is a North Carolinian and my father is a Virginian and if they taught me anything, they taught me to be polite, to everyone; so I ignored my secret desire to ask, "Why, in God's name, do you care?" and just smiled and worked it out in my head that these people were not pushy and rude, they were just trying to be nice. The pearl earrings and rotten teeth I could take, it was the question of more children that sent me running.

It might have started with our doorman or the check-out lady at the Food Emporium or an already pregnant-with-the-second mother in the park, but the question was out and running, its prize: me. There was one woman in particular, a mother of five and a grandmother of twelve, I came to learn, who lived in our building and liked to mill around the mailroom at all hours of the day. She was old, with tough, wrinkled brown skin and a tough, husky voice to match. I remember standing before my mailbox, carrying my bald and drooling daughter in a sling, unprepared for the question which came at me like a body slam. She leaned close to my daughter's face and proceeded to speak of me in the third-person, as she explained how her mommy was depriving her of siblings and what a terrible shame that was. Then she peered up at me, the guilty party, and said: "Wine. A little red wine right before your husband comes home, it always did the trick for me." I nodded obediently. The question became palpable every time my daughter and I left the apartment; I could feel its presence as we walked down the street, as we rode the bus, or waited in line for coffee; it had a heartbeat, it had a pulse, and I knew that its desire for answers was as strong as my desire to hide them, escape from each other, if possible, would be a nasty affair. In the meantime, I suppose it was that polite upbringing that helped me enact the rare art of answering a question without really answering it. I stretched, spun, disguised the truth, and sometimes I lied until that question had retreated back to its hole.

I finally told the old woman in the mailroom that I had ordered a case of red wine, then gave my husband the job of getting the mail.

Motherhood is like celebrity, and this is actually much worse than it sounds. People pretend to be bored, uninspired, even exhausted by it, and yet who has not stared at the enormous belly of a pregnant woman, or peeked inside the pram of a newborn, or studied the celebrity standing next to you at the coffee shop waiting for his cappuccino? Curiosity is expected, often harmless, within the public culture of social interactions ("How old is your daughter?" "How do you manage to get yourself, your daughter, and your stroller onto the bus?"); but when curiosity steps over the line into ownership, good manners are replaced with unbending and relentless fervor ("Your daughter is much too old for a pacifier!" "Hey, Lady, hurry up and get your kid on the bus! Jesus! You ever heard of walking?") that in a blink of an eye turns self-righteous, smug, and cruel. With motherhood and celebrity there is no line drawn, your rights to privacy vanish, and your every move, your every decision is judged and scrutinized freely. Mothers are disparaged for irresponsibility and selfishness, the same way celebrities are for growing old and fat. The idea that mothers should always be Good (as in "God is Great, God is Good" kind of good) and selfless, and celebrities should always be young and beautiful, is a fantasy that has somehow been transformed into truth. I never appreciated this before I was a mother, I never understood how heavily our society relies on such fantasies, and how quickly the poor soul who falls short of the fantasy is punished and vilified.

Up until tonight I have felt a sense of peace, a calm acceptance about my body failing on me. I have been rational, pragmatic, and at times actually cheerful in explaining to my family and closest friends that my uterus no longer works. I came up with elaborate metaphors: think of a marathon runner with a torn A.C.L., cataracts, hearing loss, lactose intolerance. We're not talking death here, we're talking about a malfunction, a glitch, what was once perfect no longer is, and never will be again — everyone can understand this, everyone can relate, I thought. I fought off their pity with optimism, their worry with encouragement, their questions with sound, medical answers. I found myself in the mysterious role of cheerleader, not in the metaphorical sense, but in the literal sense, with a permanent smile and extra high kicks. I persuaded, I explained, I campaigned for the bright side until all of the people in this small, carefully chosen group no longer looked at me with pity, curiosity, or worry. I had fought for normalcy and thought I had won.

But it is on page 68 of *Homemade Baby Food* when it all falls apart: "Don't let looks fool you. Clean-looking food, equipment, and utensils may not be sanitary." And before my eyes the author comes to life, shaking her finger at me, not because I haven't sterilized my daughter's bowls and spoons and cups (because I have, I swear), but because I cannot carry another child. I am like that pitiful mother, caught red-handed as she tries to pass off canned applesauce for the real thing. My secret will be out soon, there will be no more hiding, no more lying, no more pretending. Paying another woman to carry my baby is not natural, it isn't normal, it's cheating.

***

Throughout my childhood I did not perceive my mother as human.

A human mother was a paradox to me. Mothers were their own species, like mermaids, lovely and rare in their complete and total willingness to sacrifice every part of themselves for the goodness of their children. In my world mothers and grandmothers could cook, sew, decorate a home, arrange roses exquisitely, throw lavish parties, mix fancy drinks, deep-sea fish and pull in a blue marlin, give speeches and witty toasts, make any man comfortable, play the piano, oil paint, sketch, sculpt, and provide the deepest love and comfort a child could ever need; and smile while doing it all. If I viewed myself as the center of my mother's world, she was completely, body, mind, and soul, the center of mine. Adrienne Rich writes in *Of Woman Born*: "The first knowledge any woman has of warmth, nourishment, tenderness, security, sensuality, mutuality, comes from her mother. The earliest enwrapment of one female body with another can sooner or later be denied or rejected, felt as choking possessiveness, as rejection, trap or taboo; but it is, at the beginning, the whole world."

But then I turned thirteen, and things began to change. My mother and I had an argument, I declared my hatred of her then slammed my bedroom door in her face. I stood in my room waiting for pleas of apology, but there was only silence. Then I heard her voice: "Sometimes I don't like you either." I was shocked — and for a split second felt the victim's rush of vindication. I threw open my door, ready to punish her. But as I stood face to face with my mother and studied her expression of hurt, I finally understood the terrible truth: my mother was an actual human being.

The truth is inevitable; my grandfather calls it, "whistling by the graveyard." I have often thought about that moment when I was thirteen, right before I opened my bedroom door. What was about to happen would not only change everything between my mother and me, but it would change my view of myself and my role in the world. Somewhere inside my body of raging hormones and self-centeredness I knew the honeymoon of childhood was coming to an end, and that I would have to enter the very grown-up world of accountability; and the same clairvoyant instincts have kicked in twenty-two years later as I lie in the dark with the homemade baby food book on my chest listening to my daughter breathe through the white noise of the baby monitor. When I was thirteen there was the saving grace of other miserable thirteen-year-olds, the music of The Smiths, black eyeliner, Judy Blume, the gorgeousness of Sting to provide an escape, a refuge from confusion and adolescent inertia. Now at thirty-five I find myself alone, cast as a character in a strange story that bears no precedent. My mother and grandmothers offer no point of reference to this: an observer to one's baby growing inside another. There are no guidebooks, no models to explain why this sudden slap of shame has taken hold of me; why I look at the small black and white sonogram picture of my nine-week-old embryo and feel equal parts elation and grief; and why I cannot reconcile the gift of carrying a baby, that had been taken away from me, with the gift that I have been given.

I am here now, in a world of disconnect where I do not recognize myself, and I wasn't prepared for any of it. These two selves need to make peace; they must lie in bed together, listen to the hum of the baby monitor and somehow, through the white noise, hear music. I just need to figure out how to do it.

Two Years Earlier

First Meeting

There is a common misunderstanding among all human beings who have ever been born on the earth that the best way to live is to try and avoid pain and just try to get comfortable. You can see this even in insects and animals and birds. All of us are the same...

If we are committed to comfort at any cost, as soon as we come against the least edge of pain, we're going to run; we'll never know what's beyond that particular barrier or wall or fearful thing.

Pema Chodron, Nun of the Kagyu Order of Tibetan Buddhism

On the morning of August 17, 2003, my husband and I drive out of New York City headed for Annapolis, Maryland. We will spend the day at the office of The Center for Surrogate Parenting (CSP). In a letter from the program administrator we are told that during this four to six hour consultation we will meet with her as well as a counselor, and we will also have the opportunity to speak with a lawyer. This meeting will be our first step in the surrogacy process.

In the car I hold on my lap a notebook in which I have written intricate and detailed notes on all of the literature the agency has sent me. I study these notes, highlight portions of interest, quiz my husband. There is a different language in this world of surrogacy, in all of its literature the wording never strays from this language: the surrogate is never referred to as "the surrogate," but always as "the surrogate mother." As I read aloud the profile of a "typical surrogate mother" the tone of the profile becomes elevated:

> She can best be described as a responsible and empathetic woman who looks forward to the experience of helping an infertile couple have a child of their own. A re-occurring theme stated by surrogate mothers is that the true genesis of the child is its creation in the minds and hearts of the intended parents.

What suddenly comes to mind is the famous painting of the Virgin Mary, *Madonna and Child*, that I have seen at the Metropolitan Museum of Art.

"That sounds good," my husband says. I can always rely on him to be upbeat; of course, he is a Catholic.

"Let's move on," I say.

I explain to him that the parents of the baby-to-be are always referred to as "the couple" or "the intended mother" and "the intended father." There are different kinds of surrogacy programs: "Traditional Surrogacy" or "AI" (Artificial Insemination) in which the surrogate mother is inseminated with the sperm of the intended father; there is "IVF/ED" (In Vitro Fertilization and Egg Donation) in which ovum from a donor is fertilized with sperm from the intended father with the resulting embryos implanted into the uterus of the surrogate mother; and finally there is Gestational Surrogacy / IVF in which ovum and sperm from the couple are combined to create embryos that are implanted into the uterus of the surrogate mother; the final program, I remind my husband, is the one we will participate in.

There is also a questionnaire, which we have planned to complete during this three-hour car ride:

- Why have you chosen to pursue surrogate parenting? Have you told anyone of your plans to work with a surrogate, and if so what were their reactions? Do you need help in explaining surrogacy to a family member

or a friend?
- What qualities do you want your surrogate to have? What type of contact do you want to have with your surrogate during the pregnancy and after the birth? Will you request your surrogate undergoes an amniocentesis, and if so what will you do with the results?
- Will you elect to terminate a pregnancy if there is a diagnosis for Downs syndrome, or only for something more severe?
- Will you do selective reduction?
- What do you plan to tell the child about his/her unique origins?
- How has the struggle of infertility affected your marriage?
- How would you describe yourselves to a potential surrogate mother?
- How can we help make this a good experience for you?

I want us to be prepared, or at least appear prepared, for I understand that not only are we assessing this agency, but we too are being assessed and I want us to shine. I jot down our answers quickly, precisely, this is easier than I thought. When the counselor asks us these questions my husband and I will not hesitate, we will not look at each other blankly searching for the right answer because we now have in our possession all of the answers to every possible question; we might be the most prepared and together parents the agency has ever met.

Of course all of this carefully constructed preparedness will come crashing down on me in a year; but for now I continue to review my notes, apply make-up, and stare out the window at Annapolis, a city I had not visited since I was twelve.

What greets us in the lobby of the agency's office is a blown-up poster of the cover of *People* magazine featuring Joan Lunden and her surrogate mother; they both smile, they gush with happiness. As I study the poster I realize that I, too, am smiling as I stare at their smiles; perhaps like a cold, smiling is contagious.

But the smile on my face suddenly begins to hurt, the same way the mouth grows sore when told to smile for family pictures.

We are escorted into a room that looks like a conference room with a long table and chairs; it is comfortable and plain. My husband and I sit across from the program administrator who is soft-spoken and friendly; we show her our passports, our marriage certificate, and give her our questionnaire and check for $400 that covers the cost of this consultation. I also show her pictures of our daughter. She gives us an overview of the agency: it is the largest and oldest private agency in the world, since its beginnings in 1986 in California. The Annapolis office was opened in 1999 to make travel more convenient for couples on the east coast, as well as overseas. It is important for us to understand that surrogacy is still a grey issue in many states; in California, for example, surrogacy is unregulated, allowing anyone to start an agency and advertise willing surrogates for X amount of dollars — one can imagine the abuses such an open market invites, especially when you are dealing with desperate couples wanting a child. Theirs is the only agency that allows a couple to meet a surrogate mother only after she has passed and completed her rigorous psychological and medical screening, a process which can take up to three months.

And there is more.

This agency is the most respected in the world. A large portion of their clients are from Europe; legal surrogacy is limited in Europe, and when allowed complicated. Only the UK and Israel have legislation allowing the practice of surrogacy; though in both countries the surrogate cannot be financially compensated. In Israel, for example, legislation gives the surrogate the right to decide during the first seven days of the baby's life whether she would like to break the contract and keep the child.

A nightmare like that would never happen in this agency, she assures us.

I listen to her pitch, I nod my head, I smile when I am supposed to smile, but what is strange is how disinterested I am in the details. I am fidgety, my mind wanders, I think about lunch. I wonder if that diner is still here, the one by the marina that my brother and I would walk to in the mornings; my parents would still be asleep, but the two of us were early risers, we always wandered out to explore alone.

My mind shifts back to the room and the coordinator's voice. What I am thinking now is: sounds great, where do I sign up? I glance over at my husband. He, on the other hand, is focused and taking notes.

It is now my turn to explain to her my "medical issue," the reason why I cannot carry another baby. I relay my issues quickly as if from a script or a report, without emotion, without drama. She nods, expresses concern and disappointment for me, which makes me uncomfortable, though I understand it is her job to feel sorry for me.

"Of course we will need a letter and documents from your doctor, verifying these medical issues," she says.

"Of course."

Because we live in New York, a state that does not permit surrogacy, we will have to choose a fertility clinic in a state that does permit surrogacy, like Maryland or Virginia, for example. Their agency works closely with Shady Grove Fertility Center, which has fifteen locations in the Washington Metropolitan area. Most all of the agency's European clients use this clinic. She gives us brochures on Shady Grove and goes into greater detail on the facility and the excellent staff. I write a note to my husband on my notebook; I nudge his leg and slide the notebook toward him, as if we are in high school again: *lunch after this*? I write. He ignores me. I place the notebook back onto my lap and doodle over my message until it is nothing but a set of 8's interlocked across the page.

At the time I don't view my behavior as immature or irresponsible because the denial has already set in; to actually be present, to engage myself in the consultation, like my husband, would have been a form of acceptance that all of this was real.

The next topic of importance is the "profile letter," she explains. This will be our letter to a perspective surrogate introducing ourselves; this letter is vital, without it the process cannot move forward. We are given a handout with guidelines and tips on writing this letter:

Your profile should fill two to three pages typed and

printed on paper with an appropriate border design or other decorative element (not plain white or gray). A surrogate may receive letters and photographs on more than one couple and her decision as to which couple she chooses to assist is based on this information. Therefore, it is very important that your letter be personal, warm and detailed. Try to give her a sense of who you are, your feelings for each other and the life your child will have. Address the letter "Dear Surrogate Mother." If English is not your primary language, please call if you need help or advice.

I write down "profile letter" in my notebook and circle it, then circle it again. This will be simple; I am a writer after all. I glance down at my watch.

"Wait a minute," my husband says. "The surrogate chooses us?"

I stare at him, his tone is just a touch confrontational and I don't want this woman to think we are raving lunatics.

"Well," she begins. "Not exactly."

"But the surrogate sees our profile first, then decides if she likes us or not," he says.

"Well, yes. When a surrogate mother expresses interest in you, her profile is then sent to you. Then you and your wife decide if you think she might be a good fit or not. In the end it is a mutual decision."

As I read further down on the handout, there is a list of topics that the profile letter must cover:

- Thank you to surrogate mother for considering you.

- Names and ages *(the coordinator tells us that we should never use the pronoun "I" but always use "We" and use our names, even when describing oneself)*
- Short description of why you are requesting the help of a surrogate
- How you met, how long you have known each other, and when you were married

- Physical description, as well as personality traits, your relationship and/or outlook on life (some couples find it easier to describe each other)
- Where you each grew up and where you live now (city, suburb, apartment, single family home)
- Other children you have (names, ages, description); pets
- Extended family (parents' siblings), where they live and how much contact you expect them to have with your child
- Occupations
- Religious affiliations
- What do you do for enjoyment, hobbies, and vacations
- What kind of relationship and how much contact you would like to have with your surrogate mother both during the pregnancy and after the birth
- Thank you to surrogate mother for considering you
- **HAND-WRITTEN SIGNATURE**

All of this information must be written on no more than three pages.

We are shown samples of actual profile letters. These are not just letters, these are albums, elaborate portfolios, bound, quilted and decoupaged to the nines. We open them slowly, carefully; I feel like I am invading privacy, peeking into a stranger's underwear drawer. As specified in the profile letter tips, none of the books contains white or grey paper, there is a lot of pink and mauve paper, as well as light blue, yellow and peach. Centered on these pages are photographs, mostly of childless couples on their wedding day and honeymoon, on biking trips, beach trips, picnics in the park. All of the men and women are conspicuously without children, though many hold pets in their arms. I flip quickly through the books, smiling, commenting to the coordinator how nice they are because she is watching me; the truth is I find them depressing and sad.

My husband begins a series of questions about surrogate mothers; I take a deep breath. I sit up straight and rub the small of my back.

I feel like I want to jump out of my skin or perhaps scream.
"Who are these women?" he asks.
I stare at him with disbelief. The answer to that question was all laid out in the literature I highlighted, the literature which now the coordinator knows he did not read:

> A typical surrogate mother would be described as an empathetic, giving, kind, and healthy woman between the ages of 21-40 years old, who has 2 children and 13 years of formal education. Seventy-five percent are married and one third have full-time employment. The majority of surrogate mothers are raised in the Christian faith, with 25% raised Catholic.... The motivations to become a surrogate mother include: a) enjoy being pregnant, b) have a history of easy, uncomplicated pregnancies, c) an opportunity to feel special, d) empathy for childless couples, e) importance of their children in their lives, f) opportunity to make a unique contribution, g) financial gain for her family, and h) an opportunity to make up for a pregnancy previously terminated.

The coordinator smiles and relays pretty much the same information that was in the literature. I smile, nod my head, making it clear to her that I completely get who these women are, I did my homework; but my husband stares at her blankly.

The door opens and another woman enters the room. She is a psychological counselor, one of the many who not only screens potential surrogate mothers, but who also works as a liaison between the surrogate mother and the couple throughout IVF and the pregnancy.

I take a bathroom break. I walk down the hall, past a room, and through the space in the blinds I glimpse the backs of a man and a woman sitting side by side in over-sized chairs; a woman sits across from them. I immediately know that the man and the woman are a couple, not a couple like my husband and me, but a potential surrogate mother and her husband being interviewed for the job. I don't know how I know this, I just do.

When I return my husband and the counselor are chatting it up, something about skiing out west. She wears Birkenstocks and loose-fitting clothes, her manner is laid back, friendly, peaceful; in an emergency she would be the only calm person in the room. I immediately like her. She sits across from us with an expression of complete empathy. She sees through our smiles something I don't even see yet.

"Tell me about your daughter," she begins.

The question is brilliant, it not only undermines awkward moments at cocktail parties, but it works in surrogacy consultations as well. I immediately feel my shoulders relax, I begin to breathe normally; I no longer want to kill my husband. He, too, is suddenly more relaxed, he smiles as we talk about our girl. The counselor gradually leads us back to why we are here. She, too, describes a typical surrogate mother profile, which is exactly like the one the coordinator had described but, as if already anticipating my husband's uncertainty, she elaborates, explaining in greater detail her job of screening potential surrogates, meeting their spouses and always knowing within the first five minutes of a meeting if the woman's motivation is money or a higher purpose.

"Money is never the driving incentive with our surrogate mothers," she explains. "There are plenty of agencies out there recruiting women who simply want a paycheck. But we have found that money is never a healthy reason, for anyone."

"If not for money, then why do the women you choose want to do this?" My husband asks. I stare at him and wonder why he didn't bring this question up in the car, the answer was in the literature.

The counselor goes on to describe the typical surrogate mother as a wife, a mother of three school-aged children, a "soccer mom" who wants to do something for the greater good. She carries babies easily and would like to share the gift of family with a couple who has not had the good fortune of having children, as she has had. Of course the money is nice because this woman often puts it toward her children's college education or toward their savings, or to help out with the mortgage. In the end, everybody wins.

My husband's expression is still incredulous.

I would like to interject that even in a "normal" situation men have a difficult time grasping the physicality and the desire of carrying a child, but the idea of another woman, a stranger, volunteering her body to carry a child for people whom she doesn't know just might be impossible for a man to ever truly grasp; and I am slowly realizing that perhaps I don't fully grasp it either. But now that my husband has revealed his anxiety to the counselor, my job is to appear completely together, completely cognizant of what we are getting ourselves into, so I say nothing and continue taking notes.

"Will there be some kind of prejudice against us — since we already have a child?" my husband asks.

The counselor is careful. "No, I don't believe so. But I also think you shouldn't make your daughter the main focus of your profile letter. One picture of her will be sufficient."

I write this down.

My husband is curious about the counselor's role: *the liaison between the surrogate mother and couple* — what does that mean? She gives us an example of a common issue.

"Let's say a surrogate mother is 32 weeks pregnant and she wants to attend her 15th high school reunion, but the reunion is in Florida and she lives in Ohio. The couple does not feel comfortable with her flying at this stage in the pregnancy, even though the doctor says it is fine, and they don't want to upset their surrogate mother by telling her not to go — so they call me, and we figure out a solution."

"So what would the solution be?" My husband asks. "She shouldn't go to the reunion." He actually sounds angry.

I take a deep breath. He has done it now. In our file there will be a big black X over our names.

The counselor smiles and nods her head; she has seen his kind before.

"I agree with you," she says. "But I can assure you that we always come to a fair agreement. None of our surrogate mothers would ever do anything to endanger the babies or upset the couple."

I believe her. In fact, I would like her to handle everything. I am ready at this moment to sign off all my responsibilities to her because this lady gets it, she will take care of everything and I can go back to New York and not worry about a thing.

"So you will be our counselor," I say.

"Not necessarily," she replies. "It will depend on who you are matched with. Each counselor is assigned different surrogate mothers, so maybe you will be matched with one of mine; or maybe not." The color must have disappeared from my face because she adds, "I would love to handle your case, but all the counselors here are wonderful. You will be in good hands." Then she quickly changes the subject.

"Have you discussed what you intend to tell your child in the future? About his or her unique beginnings?" she asks.

My husband and I stare at each other blankly.

This had been a question on the questionnaire. It had been a question that had actually stumped us in the car because it had hit a nerve. What I had written on the questionnaire was: *honesty is the best policy*! A safe, non-committal answer. But the truth was we didn't have a set answer, certainly not one that would neatly fill the two lines of the questionnaire. The question carries with it all sorts of strange scenarios and possible outcomes that neither of us wanted to deal with in the car that morning, nor does it appear we want to deal with now, sitting opposite the counselor who patiently awaits our answer.

The problem is not that we do not have an answer, but that our answer is convoluted, perhaps even inappropriate for this meeting. What I do not feel comfortable revealing to her is my feeling that no parent wants their child deemed as "different." I would argue that point even outside our homogenous culture. What you hope for your child is an even playing field, at least in the beginning. Our second child has not even been born, and yet already her beginnings are different. How can I possibly imagine what I will say to this unborn child years from now about his or her "unique beginnings," when I barely have a grip on them myself?

I cannot relay to this woman my husband's fear that this child might forever be defined as a "surrogate baby;" or my reply, "that it won't matter, how he or she got here simply won't matter," meaning, perhaps, that the topic need never come up.

What we experienced in the car that morning was fear of the unknown, the fear of embracing differences, the fear of accepting one's lot and forging ahead.

The reality is we both knew our answer to that question; we both knew what we would some day tell this child: *honesty is the best policy*, of course, without the smug write-off. We just weren't ready to rehearse for it yet.

I now feel the counselor's eyes on me.

"Do you have any questions?" I shake my head no. But then my husband takes a deep breath and finally asks the question that has been bothering him all morning.

"How do we know this woman won't want our baby?" he asks.

The fact that his question sounds like the title of a movie on Lifetime Television for Women is less shocking to me than the counselor's reaction: she sort of laughs. No, it's not really a laugh, it is a cross between a sound in her throat that translates to something like, *ahh*, combined with a smile. She has obviously heard this question hundreds of times. She looks at my husband and nods her head like she understands completely.

"Surrogate mothers do not want your baby," she says.

Her voice is one of compassion, with a nice dose of practicality. The agency provides its surrogate mothers a counseling service in the form of group meetings, in which surrogate mothers gather together over a weekend and participate in a retreat of sorts, talking about their experiences, exchanging stories, seeking advice, etc. The counselor tells us that that particular question always gets laughs out of the surrogate mothers because as much as they adore children, the last thing they want is your baby; they have their own children and are well past the diapers and bottles stage; they don't want to go back.

I smile, nodding my head along with the counselor to let her know that I understand, that I am on the same page as her, and that my husband — he's only a man, after all — just needs a little reassurance, a little hand-holding, and that I will take care of him,

I will ease his mind. Through the blinds on the window I can see just part of the poster of Joan Lunden and her surrogate mother hanging in the lobby; look how happy they are, look how kind her surrogate mother appears, she doesn't look like a psychopath.

When the counselor departs we are left alone to speak to a lawyer in California, via speaker phone, who specializes in surrogacy law. His law firm is one most of the couples in this agency use, and because his law firm is not employed by The Center for Surrogate Parenting Agency, and because he works with other surrogacy agencies, he can be objective in answering my husband's questions as to why this agency is the best. Aside from the agency's excellent reputation and longevity and impressive birth rates, Dr. Hannah Burns, is the main reason, in his opinion, why CSP is the best. Dr. Burns is the head of the counseling staff, she has been involved in evaluating surrogate mothers and helping couples for 25 years. I read in the literature that "she is recognized as a world-renowned leader in the psychological evaluation of surrogate mothers." She is the backbone of the agency, he adds.

We should also understand that our surrogate mother will not reside in New York. New York surrogacy laws are impossible: it is illegal for a surrogate to be financially compensated for carrying a baby.

"But we can fly her to New York to give birth," I say. "So we can use my doctor." I look at my husband, at least the baby can be born at New York Presbyterian, like our daughter.

That is out of the question, he tells us. No part of the surrogacy arrangement can take place in New York, not the IVF transfer of embryos, nor the birth. The baby will be born in whatever state the surrogate mother resides.

How did I miss that detail in the literature?

It wasn't in the literature.

I stare at my husband.

"What about Connecticut?" my husband asks.

Connecticut is tricky as well. If we should find a surrogate mother in Connecticut we would have to re-adopt the baby in New York (my husband and I exchange a glance, that is out of the question), so perhaps it is best to stay away from Connecticut.

The most surrogacy friendly states are Ohio, Illinois, California, of course, just to name a few.

"I know that's not exactly convenient for you," the lawyer says. "But neither is this whole arrangement."

He has ended the phone call with the understatement of the day.

When we leave the office and step into the streets of Annapolis, I feel dizzy. Five hours we have spent in the office of the surrogate agency; I shade my eyes from the bright afternoon sunlight. We walk down the cobble-stoned streets of the city. The sun is setting over the Chesapeake. We walk past the marina and I point to the exact dock where we used to dock my father's boat when my brother and I were kids, it is hard to believe that I remember this, but I do.

I would like to have dinner at that diner where my brother and I used to go, but as we walk to find it I see that it is gone, the building has been torn down and replaced by a parking garage.

So we eat ice cream for dinner, walk a little more, then get in our car and drive back to New York.

March 8, 2005

A Match

Dear Mr. and Mrs. Dyson,

Greetings! Enclosed is information on a potential surrogate mother that I would like for you to consider. I am the counselor who did Norah's initial interview. Norah has been a surrogate mother before. Therefore, if you select Norah as your surrogate mother, I would work with you throughout your relationship with her.

Sincerely,

Rachel O'Clair
MFCC

Dear Intended Parent,

Welcome to CSP and to your journey into parenthood. My name is Norah. I am 37, and a single mom to 3 boys. I have been very fortunate and grateful to have helped two other couples become a family. Morgan was born in 1998, and Adam was born in 2002. I had never thought about becoming a surrogate more than once, but when I saw the look on the faces of Morgan's parents when she entered the world, I knew I wanted to help another couple. The birth of Adam was just as special. His parents were by my side to greet him and the room was filled with joyful tears. I feel that since I am healthy and still able to help another couple, it would be selfish of me not to. Surrogacy will always be in my heart. I have met the most wonderful and amazing people and some very special friends through surrogacy.

I grew up with two older brothers and had a great childhood. My father passed away when I was only 2 from a work accident and my mom raised the three of us on her own. I have great respect for her and believe my independence and drive is from her and her strength to overcome obstacles life sometimes brings, to push forward, make the most of what you have and enjoy life to the fullest. She is a little old fashioned, but has always supported me and my decisions. I have been single for almost two years now and the boys have a great relationship with their father. Some day I would like to find the right person and get married again, but for now, I am just enjoying being a mom to the boys and trying to keep up with them. I would have to say my favorite hobby is photography. I love to capture great pictures and keep telling myself that I am going to take some classes, but I haven't seemed to get around to that yet. I love to do activities with my boys. We do everything from baseball games, amusement parks, hiking, monster truck shows, football games, picnicking, to anything outdoors, bike riding, horseback riding, going to the movies. Just about the only thing I don't really enjoy is camping, but the boys love it so I manage to rough it for them. We also love to travel and go to new places and learn new things. We usually have a great time no matter where we go or what we do.

I am very proud of all three boys and love being a mom to them. It is however, not an easy job sometimes. It is so rewarding for me to watch them grow, learn, and accomplish new things. It is also a major headache when they can't seem to get along, and all want to go in different directions.

I can't wait to help another couple feel all of these joys. Being a parent is the best and I hope that I can help someone else become a parent and join them with the miracle of having a healthy, bouncing baby to love and enjoy. If you choose me to help complete your family, I look forward to meeting you and learning more about you. If I am not the right surrogate mother for you, I wish you the best on your journey.
Sincerely,
Norah

***

I meet Norah for the first time at Reagan National Airport on April 21, 2005. Tomorrow we have our first meeting with the fertility doctor at Shady Grove Fertility Center in Maryland. They will do blood work on Norah and map out the plan for the next few months. The aim here is to match Norah's menstrual cycle with mine, as well as to set up a time line for progesterone shots, which Norah will give herself, in order to prepare her uterus for embryo implantation.

I am alone inside the terminal, standing a few feet away from a small group of people also waiting. My husband is waiting in the car outside. It smells like doughnuts, and my heart is racing. I hold a small bouquet of flowers that, now on closer inspection, seem completely inadequate; I should have brought chocolates. But what if she's allergic to chocolate? No, I should have gone for jewelry, earrings or a bracelet would have been better, small hoops or a handsome, gold bracelet with a charm, a charm with her initials engraved on it; I remember from her pictures that Norah wore gold. Or perhaps that would have been too much, I don't want to scare her. A scarf would have been nice, but maybe she's not the scarf type; or a pretty candle? But if it broke in her luggage that would be a mess. Hand lotion, guest soap, potpourri. I stare down at the flowers, in the middle of the pink roses is a small, pathetic carnation that has begun to wilt. I pull it out and toss it in the trash. The bouquet will have to do.

A crowd of people who have just de-planed are walking toward us. I have seen Norah only in the pictures that she sent. And now here she is. Her smile is radiant. She is much shorter than me, she looks like a gymnast, strong with great posture. We embrace and begin to talk as if we are old friends, as if this isn't one of the strangest arrangements in the history of humankind.

First Trimester

Identity Crisis...the concept deals with the relationship between what a person appears to be in the eyes of others and what he or she feels he or she is. It refers to the dynamics of the search for an inner continuity that will match the external social conditions....

In short, [adolescence] means social existence without a clear blueprint for behavior.

Hans Sebald, *Adolescence: A Social Psychological Analysis*

Norah is 13 weeks pregnant today. The baby is about 3 inches long and its face is beginning to look more human. The eyes have moved closer together and the ears lie flat, though they have not quite made it to the side of the head. Fingerprints are already formed and it's starting to urinate amniotic fluid. Norah feels good, though she can no longer lie on her stomach comfortably. She has the feeling it's a boy, but we're not going to find out.

I have a sixteen-year-old brother. He embodies many of the characteristics that our society has deemed "adolescent." He is moody, withdrawn, confused, unpredictable, irrational, and self-conscious; he practices bad hygiene and possesses equally bad taste in clothes; he and his friends formed a band, though none of them play an instrument. When we visit my family I observe in him moments of childlike delight and innocence, recognizing the boy whom I used to carry on my hip, the boy whom I adored; but as quickly as a smile graces his face, something between a frown and an expression of indifference inevitably replaces it, revealing this new boy-man who has suddenly developed a hearing problem and just wants to be left alone. When I look to my mother for help, for some explanation, for a solution to make him *normal* again, she only raises her eyebrows at me. So I take matters into my own hands: I bribe him. I give him cash; I drive him and his girlfriend to the movies; I drive them to Wal-Mart at ten o'clock at night; I give him more cash. And as a last resort I take him to dinner at McDonald's. We sit across from each other in a bright, orange booth. It is after 9 pm and the place is empty, save for the manager who is taking his break at a small table for two by the front window. There is an eeriness to this quiet, to the buzzing fluorescent lights overhead, to the abandoned play yard outside and the absence of background music; even the deep fryers have been turned off for the night. My brother slouches over his Big Mac and Supersize fries and strawberry milkshake; I sip Diet Coke. I study his long, unwashed hair, the line of small red pimples running along his forehead and chin, his bony fingers and broad, sharp shoulders, his square jaw and blue eyes. I can feel how he savors the silence, with each bite praying his annoying sister will keep her mouth shut and let him eat in peace. He doesn't want to answer any more of her impossible questions: How's school? What do you want to do with your life? Why don't you want to play checkers? You used to love checkers. What's wrong with you? Why are you so changed?

Finally he looks up at me, he can bear it no more: *What!* It is more an exclamation than a question, and I can see on his face that he is just as confused and exhausted with his life as an adolescent as I am, but this is where he is now and there is nothing he can do about it. He lets out a deep sigh, then retreats back to his meal.

I lean back in the booth and feel my shoulders relax. The tension I have felt in my body for months now softens as I understand something horrible but somehow wonderfully true: I know exactly how he feels. Like him, I find myself suspended in an ambiguous and scary place, dodging unanswerable questions, deflecting criticism, feigning deafness; I, too, am plagued with self-doubt, powerlessness, vicious mood swings, and a bit of acne; like him, I would very much like to hide from the world. I want to reach across the table and hug and kiss him; for a moment I feel the euphoria, the utter relief, of having finally found someone who speaks my language.

I watch him lick catsup and grease off his fingers, then wipe his hands on his jeans before returning to his Big Mac. The euphoria is gone as I stand up and walk to get him some napkins. Words like "pig" and "barnyard" race through my mind as I sit back down and set a large pile of napkins neatly in front of him, none of which does he bother to use. I tell myself to let it alone, but I cannot help it, and just as I open my mouth to ask whether he has forgotten about the manners our mother tirelessly taught him, or if he just prefers to eat like a pig, music blasts from somewhere. I feel myself jump. It is a rap song, a man's voice shouts from the speakers, his anger elevated by an edgy, sharp electronic beat. The manager is up now, hurrying back to the kitchen. There is a commotion, we hear voices and laughter as the music suddenly stops, and all is quiet again. I look at my brother, he peers up at me; in spite of ourselves, we smile.

The only book on surrogacy that I can find is one the agency recommended — it is a children's book about a couple named Sandy and Bob who have a cat named Pancake and a dog named Spot, and they dream of having a baby. I am not that desperate yet, so I buy Erik H. Erikson's, *Identity: Youth and Crisis.* When my three-year-old strolls into my office (located next door to her bedroom) I turn the book over in order to hide its title, as if she can read. Immediately sensing that I am hiding something from her, she grabs the book from my desk and scurries into her room, slamming the door behind her. I open the door to find her lounging on her small toddler bed flipping through the book, reciting the alphabet. When I ask her to give me the book she ignores me and continues to turn the pages, wrinkling her brow in deep concentration. When I insist, and the tone of my voice shifts to one of irritation, she holds her finger up to me and pierces her lips together; I immediately retreat and imagine my girl years from now in therapy because her mother wouldn't let her read books about therapy. For the next week she carries the book around the apartment, slips it safely into her backpack, and insists on taking it to bed with her. When we have visitors I rush to hide the book in my closet, and feign ignorance when she asks after its whereabouts. It is so strange how she won't move on from her fixation with Erikson's book. There are no pictures, only the small black and white photo of Erikson himself on the cover, looking pensive and tired the way a wise person who possesses all of life's answers should look. She watches me closely, studies my reaction as she parades the book around; I pretend that I no longer want it, but somehow she knows better.

There is something motherly as well as childlike in her insistence to keep the book away from me. By making it her own she is, in a sense, attempting to control whatever it is lurking within the pages that makes my forehead wrinkle and my smile disappear. But this ownership also rings of anger, she does not want me to read this book and scribble in the margins anymore, she does not want me to disappear in thought; she wants me, without the book, back. I believe she is trying to protect me and punish me all at once.

> For no matter what we do in detail, the child will primarily feel what it is we live by as loving, co-operative, and firm beings, and what makes us hateful, anxious, and divided in ourselves.

What Erikson writes is painfully true. When I sigh in exasperation my daughter sighs too; when I argue with my husband my daughter paces the room and mimics our voices; when I am overcome with impatience and resort to breathing exercises that never work, my daughter touches my arm gently and asks, "Are you happy?" Lying to my daughter is like lying to myself, it is a constant battle that can only be won by coming clean. But here again, it is impossible for me to explain to her my predicament. She met Norah back in August and we explained to her that Norah would help us give her a baby sister or a baby brother; I remember how she stared at my husband and me and nodded her head, as if she understood perfectly. She understands that babies grow in bellies. She apparently has been host to two babies in her own belly since July (when I began my drug treatment for IVF). She has named them Sam and Sam, and she tells everyone, friends and strangers alike, that she has two babies in her belly. What I do not anticipate is how her innocent declaration begins to turn the light back on me. In the check-out line at the grocery store strangers peer up at me knowingly after hearing my daughter's good news: "When are you due?" they ask and wink. I glance down at my daughter, my traitor, as they wait for an answer, studying the dumbfounded look on my face. Then they add, "Is it twins?" I can see from their faces that they are hoping it is. But no, it is not twins, and no, I am not pregnant. Clearly they are disappointed.

At my daughter's pre-school there is an Open House for prospective parents. I volunteer. Since I am a new mother I am given menial tasks such as holding doors open and keeping cookie plates filled. Last spring an article came out on Bloomberg informing us that admission into Manhattan pre-schools was more competitive than Harvard's: in Manhattan there were on average 15 applicants for each spot in about 200 preschools, compared to Harvard's 11 applicants competing for each of its 2,030 spots. According to the U.S. Census, in 2003 New York had 555,526 children under the age of 5, the biggest population among U.S. cities. Our application process began last fall, which entailed school tours, lectures, interviews, and essays. Along with dozens of other prospective parents at open houses, we were herded down narrow hallways into tiny classrooms, told to sit in tiny chairs, crowded into lecture halls where directors preached about the importance of the right pre-school, vital developmental milestones that your child must achieve, lest he be doomed to a life of mediocrity and sloth, and showed adorable videos and slides of the most brilliant toddlers on earth.

At the present Open House, parents file in through the door, name-tagged and nervous. The mood is intense, naturally; this is New York City, and what we've got here is an undercroft crowded with highly-charged mothers and fathers shopping for the perfect pre-school for their kids. I notice that at least a dozen of the women are pregnant. As I watch them walk by I do not feel at all uncomfortable; I feel quite the opposite. Norah is 13 weeks pregnant now, the baby has a strong heartbeat, she has safely passed into the second trimester, there is reason to celebrate. And yet, amidst the exchange of smiles and hellos with these strangers, this excitement is replaced by a sudden urge to escape as I overhear small-talk that turns into full-blown discussions on the same theme: *When are you due? How many children do you have? Are you planning on having more? Where do your older children go to school? Was that your first choice? Are you planning on having more children? Three is the new two, you know!* I feel my body begin to inch away from the pack, afraid one of those questions will be directed at me. What will I say? Do I lie, or do I tell them the truth? Strangers are not safe, especially New Yorkers who happen to be parents; they are inquisitive and merciless in their desire to know. I make no eye contact and begin to sweat as I realize that seconds ago I felt as if I were among my peers, but now I find myself alone.

"The social scientist looks at the adolescent as going through a period of ambiguous role expectations," the sociologist Hans Sebald writes.

> The young individual often cannot decide whether a situation calls for acting as a child or as an adult, and he or she frequently suffers uncertainty in relation to the adult world—the Establishment, as it is scornfully called. This confusion does not arise in relation to his or her peer group. In fact, adolescents evade uncertainty through involvement in the group activities of their agemates and by relying on the standards of the peer group, hence forming a teenage society estranged from the larger society.

Sebald's description of the *Establishment* is for me, a thirty-five-year-old woman, my daughter's preschool (good God!), and my agemates, my peer group with whom I may form an estranged society? It does not exist.

I walk home with a friend, a safe friend. She comments on the number of pregnant women at the Open House and how she kept thinking of me.

"Because you are pregnant," she says. "You do realize that you are, right?"

I make a sound in my throat that leaves my answer open to interpretation. But the truth is, I don't. I'm not. The state of pregnancy is not an ambiguous one. You either are or you aren't. Yes, there is a baby to be sure, formed with my egg and my husband's sperm, growing inside the womb of a woman who is not me. I look the word pregnant up in the dictionary: "human pregnancy refers to the process by which a human female carries a live offspring from conception until childbirth." Clearly, I do not fall under this definition. Then I look up the word *mother*: "1. used as a title or form of address for a senior nun in a religious community; 2. used as a title of respect for a woman past middle age." There is more: "1. a woman who has a child or a female animal that has produced young; 2. a woman who acts as the parent of a child to whom she has not given birth." But the definition of 'mother' that I find most fascinating, and irrelevant, is a "slimy mass of bacteria and yeast cells that forms on the surface of alcohol being converted into acetic acid. It is added to wine cider to make vinegar; also called mother of vinegar." A slimy mass of bacteria is closer to how I feel, than pregnant. Finally I look up *surrogate:* "a woman who bears a child for a couple, with the intention of handing it over after the birth." *Handing it over?* As if it were something stolen or swiped, finally being returned to its rightful owner.

I look through my surrogate agency records to find a better definition. I find a booklet entitled, "Creating Your Family." The cover is a photograph of two hands touching, a father's and a child's, superimposed on a haze of purple, blue and pink that looks similar to depictions of heaven that I have seen in religious books and in cartoons. The folder, in which the booklet came, is decorated with purple stars and the quote: *Where Dreams Can Come True.* Inside the folder there are more purple stars encircling the name of the agency.

I open to the first page of the booklet, it reads: "Bill and I thank you for requesting our informational booklet."

Who's Bill? I read further and discover that Bill is one of the agency's directors (it is all coming back to me now). The first part of the booklet is a sales pitch, a recruitment letter of sorts, littered with exclamations and questions which Bill and his colleagues conveniently answer for you:

> Do we get more personal service with a 'smaller' program than with yours? No! Do couples report a change in their feelings about surrogacy once they become parents? *Yes! A common surprise reported by most couples was the desire to 'let the world know.'*

And there are gentle warnings against the competing surrogate agencies: "An agency claiming to have been in the practice of surrogacy for many years is probably s-t-r-e-t-c-h-i-n-g its credentials…Be careful and compare!"

I re-read the part about couples feeling overwhelmed with the desire to "let the world know" about their experience with surrogacy. Like how? With bumper stickers *(Surrogate Baby On Board)?* A newspaper ad? T-shirts? Instead of *Little Brother* or *Daddy's Girl* stenciled on those kitschy baby onesies, *Surrogate Baby* would be stenciled instead?

The agency supplies a psychological team and a staff who wear pagers. One particular member of the team "will be your new best friend, and understand[s] what you are going through." I circle this quote, as a reminder to avoid this particular member. The rest of the booklet is filled with more exclamations, stars, roses and bows, happy faces, a recommended reading list, and testimonials from surrogates and couples alike who have shared in the most wonderful "journey" of their lives.

Before I began my freshman year in college, there was a two-day retreat for new students at a place called Camp Friendship. I remember reading the description of this two-day excursion filled with terms such as "team building," "group unity," "rope courses," and "sing-a-longs," and I refused to go. What I disliked then and what I still dislike now is the notion of being grouped together with strangers who, on paper, share the same problem or circumstance; be it a bunch of 18-year olds living away from home for the first time with free access to beer, or a bunch of couples trying to have a baby. The thought of sitting around in a circle of strangers trading stories, fears, laughter and tears makes my chest and neck break out in a red rash; in fact, I feel the heat of a rash coming on at this moment just thinking about it.

Though I successfully eluded Camp Friendship as an eighteen-year-old, its counterpart awaited me, seventeen years later, in the form of the waiting room at the Shady Grove Fertility Clinic in Rockville, Maryland which I visited every day for two weeks in August in the hopes that I could grow good quality eggs. Blood monitoring and ultrasounds were done between the hours of 7 and 9:45 in the morning, and whether you arrived at 6:55 or 8:55, the room was packed with women and a handful of men. Something strange happens in the waiting room of a fertility clinic as the people file in with their Starbuck's coffees and bagels: the place transforms into something oddly reminiscent of a single's bar. First off, children are not allowed in the waiting room, this is stated many times in the clinic's booklet, and names are rarely exchanged because names are irrelevant. What defines you now is your infertility problem; what makes you interesting is just how severe or bizarre your problem is. Conversation-starters begin with eye contact and a slight smile, then the ice-breaking question: Is this your first time? The answer to this question opens up myriad discussions and immediately establishes social hierarchies: veterans vs. first-timers; success stories vs. failures; good doctor stories vs. creepy doctor stories; the nurse known as 'Jack the Ripper' vs. the nurse known as 'Nice 'n Easy.'

Apparently the waiting room is divided into sections: there is the "social section" located in the corner, loud voices and laughter burst from this corner and nurses often appear with their fingers pressed to their lips when things get a little too rowdy. There is the "quiet section" in the opposite corner with straight-back armchairs and a magazine rack; people here make no eye contact, some wear sunglasses, they slouch in their chairs and never look up from *Travel and Leisure* or *InStyle*. And finally there is the "floating section," close to the front desk, where the new patients stand nervously awaiting an empty seat. What the new patients do not yet understand is the social dynamics of the room: by sheer luck the fortunate ones will find themselves in the section where they feel most comfortable, while the not-so-fortunate ones will find themselves exactly where they do not want to be, right smack in the middle of quiet hell or social hell.

It is no coincidence that if a delusional person roaming through the New York City subway is going to pick out one person on the jam-packed train to befriend, it will be me. I don't know why this is, perhaps it goes back to that polite upbringing. It has happened often enough to lend some legitimacy to the fact that I seem to always attract the mentally disturbed, the lonely, and the talkers. Little mystery then as to where I ended up my first morning at the clinic. The empty chair in the middle of social hell is like the eye of the storm. But the danger is not located in the eye of a storm, the eye is a relatively quiet place, it is what surrounds the eye that causes the problems: the "eyewall," a ring of towering thunderstorms that causes the most destruction and severity when a cyclone hits. I have barely sat down before the questions come at me, one after another, from every direction: is this your first time? Where do you live? Do you have children? Was your daughter an IVF baby? Are those pants J. Crew? Who's your doctor? What medications are you taking? Needle in the stomach or thigh? Do you have an egg problem or a sperm problem? How many embryos do you plan to put back in? Three is the new two, you know.

I look down at my watch, it isn't even 7 am yet.

With the exception of the J. Crew pants (they are the City-Fit in dark fog), I respond to every one of their questions with half-truths. My one-word, uninspiring answers curb their initial frenzy over new blood. I think I have succeeded in convincing them that there is nothing extraordinary about my case: I am just another thirty-something with a kid, trying for another one.

But then comes another question.

"Wait, you said you live in New York City — why are you doing IVF here? New York has one of the best clinics in the country — Cornell, run by that big-wig fertility doctor, right?"

And now the group has re-focused their attention on me. I did not anticipate this follow-up question. I am not a morning person, but have found myself surrounded by chatty, relentless, morning people who have proven to be quick on their feet. My reflexes, both body and mind, are still half-asleep and I am now forgetting what exactly I have just told them.

As the group awaits my answer I stare at their expressions, curious and wanting, and realize something about "the mob" that I had never understood before: none of this questioning or prying has anything to do with me, personally, it has everything to do with information, or more precisely their fear of not possessing the *right* information. Perhaps this new person in the J. Crew pants knows something that they don't know; something important, some vital secret to having a baby. If that is the case, they will cross every line of socially accepted behavior to get me to confess everything. For them, the ends justify the means: honoring privacy is out of the question, they want answers at any cost.

But I have no answers, no secrets to share, and this is the truth.

I want to be near family while going through IVF, I tell them, to help me with my daughter, that's why I came down here. I shrug my shoulders.

The nurse calls my name.

I find the doctor's examining room with the paper dressing gown folded neatly across the stirrups oddly inviting. The boxes of plastic gloves and the tubes of KY-Jelly, the shelves of sharp instruments sealed in plastic, the boxes of condoms, and the nurse with her wide hips and tired eyes who doesn't care who I am or why I'm here, she just wants me to undress, lie down, and move my ass closer to the edge of the table — *closer, nope, closer, don't be shy, closer, that's it* — I find it all a welcome refuge. I stare at the ceiling, listen to the door open, watch the lights switch off, and now darkness, save for the glowing yellow light of the computer screen. The doctor inserts the wand between my legs, mumbles to himself, jots down numbers, negotiates the wand to the left, to the right; and now the lights are on and he has vanished. The nurse tells me to come back tomorrow as she prepares the room for the next patient. *Thank you,* I say to her as I get dressed, *Thank you.* She has no idea how much her indifference means to me.

The next morning I stand in the floating section, next to a pillar, with my face buried in a book. And for the next two weeks I stand in the same place, afraid to even sit down in the quiet section.

I sit here writing this and suddenly feel a warmth toward the women in the social corner. Yes, they were pushy and nosy, but they were not unkind. They had created this strange sisterhood of rolling members in the waiting room who shared information, advice and personal stories perhaps because that was how they survived the uncertainty and helplessness of sitting in a fertility clinic day after day. They were so open about their infertility, their husband's low sperm count, their miscarriages, their desperation for a child; there was no shame in their honesty, no bitterness, just a need to tell. I wonder what happened to the woman who was on her fifth try for a baby, or the woman who had suffered seven miscarriages, or the woman who had one child and simply wanted one more. I never knew their names, but I can see their faces. Thinking about them now, I wonder how they were able to trust others with their deepest fears and desires; where did their overriding belief in the goodness of strangers to listen, to comfort, to relate, come from? And did that goodness actually help?

When I talk to my assigned counselor, who calls me every few weeks because it is her job to do so, it is awkward.

How are things? She asks.

Great! I reply.

How is Norah?

Great!

Everything seems to be going smoothly, she says.

Yes, it does!

It is awkward because I apparently have no issues, no anxiety, and no trace of being human.

Shame, writes Erikson,

> is an infantile emotion insufficiently studied because in our civilization it is so early and easily absorbed by guilt. Shame supposes that one is completely exposed and conscious of being

looked at—in a word, self-conscious. One is visible and not ready to be visible; that is why in dreams of shame we are stared at in a condition of incomplete dress, in night attire, "with one's pants down." Shame is early expressed in an impulse to bury one's face or sink, right then and there, into the ground.

Gender Neutral Birds

Dear Mr. and Mrs. Dyson:
This letter will confirm our representation of both of you for the purpose of obtaining an agreed order of parentage and custody for the child you are expecting in April. It is our intent to obtain, if possible, an order of paternity and maternity so that the child's birth certificate will show both of you as its parents, rather than the surrogate, as you both are the genetic parents of this child. We appreciate the opportunity to work with you, and thank you for retaining our firm to handle this important matter.

Janet Alexander, Van Fleet & McHenry, Attorney at Law

The best case scenario, we are told, is that a judge will look over our contractual agreement with Norah and grant us an order of parentage and custody so that my name, and not Norah's name, will appear on the birth certificate. The worst case scenario is that the judge will deny this request, thereby leaving Norah's name on the birth certificate until I adopt the baby in New York.

There are no federal laws regulating surrogacy in the United States, and only 25 states and Washington DC have laws that even address it. Looking at the different states' laws is a bit like looking through the classifieds. Arizona, for example, prohibits surrogacy; in California surrogacy is legal and contracts are enforceable. In Washington DC all surrogacy contracts have been declared unenforceable and have been banned, violators are subject to a fine and or prison; whereas Illinois has become one of the most progressive states after the Gestational Surrogacy

Act was passed in January 2005, which states that when a child is born through gestational surrogacy the intended parents have sole custody upon the child's birth, allowing intended parents to avoid the entire adoption process, and prevents the surrogate from stating a legal claim to the baby. In Indiana surrogacy is permitted, but the state does not find surrogacy contracts enforceable (this makes no sense to me); in Florida, New Hampshire and Virginia state law limits the practice of surrogacy to infertile couples. In New York commercial surrogacy is illegal, violating this law may result in fines and possible imprisonment, but in Tennessee the state recognizes intended parents in surrogacy agreements as legal parents. And my personal favorite: Georgia, where surrogacy is neither legal nor illegal.

Even less comforting in this world of surrogacy is the name Steven Litz. On the American Surrogacy Center website I read about Indiana's surrogacy law and Litz is the author of the website's explanation of this law. He describes the law passed in 1988 which "declared surrogate contracts to be against public policy, and prohibits a court from considering a contract as a basis for determining custody in the event the surrogate refuses to give up the child." The law itself does not worry me, it is Litz's follow-up interpretation that gives me pause. He writes: "That law is basically irrelevant for two reasons: 1) in the majority of cases, the surrogate and the couple are not both from Indiana, and therefore the law does not apply, and 2) surrogacy rarely fails, so the enforcement of the contract is not an issue at all." I feel as if I am reading an adverb-laden advertisement from a smiling, mustached malpractice lawyer on the back of a Yellow Pages. He goes on to assure us that surrogacy is not outlawed in Indiana, he simply warns that if both the surrogate and the couple are from Indiana, and if the surrogate asserts legal claim of the baby, then the contract cannot be used as evidence in court. But, "in a custody fight a couple has never lost (except once where a surrogate delivered twins, the husband of the couple, incredibly, wanted only the girl, and the surrogate refused to split up the children)."

Who are these people?

When I speak to our lawyer about our case she tells us that

judges in Indiana are beginning to look at surrogacy cases with more scrutiny because of the Steven Litz case — there he is again, *Steven Litz*. It turns out that Litz is not only a lawyer, but he is also the director of a surrogate agency, Surrogate Mothers, Inc. in Monrovia, Indiana; coincidentally the same agency where Norah had signed on as a surrogate for the first time back in the 90's. Litz and his company are being investigated by a U.S. Attorney to determine whether they committed fraud or violated federal laws against child selling.

I read an article in the *Fort Wayne Journal Gazette* about the case, written on August 3, 2005. Through Litz's company, Surrogate Mothers, Inc., Stephen F. Melinger, a 58-year-old, unmarried New Jersey school teacher, hired Zaria Nkoya Huffman to bear his children through artificial insemination. The article does not state Huffman's state of residence, but she traveled to Indianapolis where she gave birth to twin girls on April 8; Melinger adopted them on April 29th. Indiana law prohibits nonresidents from adopting in Indiana, and in Melinger's court documents he claims he was an Indiana resident, listing his address as a hotel; though his driver's license lists a New Jersey address and his job is in New Jersey. And "according to court records, Melinger showed up at the hospital, where the twins were in intensive care, with a live bird in his pocket on one occasion and had bird feces on his shirt during another visit."

The twin girls were placed in foster care in May.

I find that there is a National Coalition Against Surrogacy. Jeremy Rifkin, the former chairman, is quoted in the article as saying, 'There's a difference between willingly taking someone's baby and carrying it as a token of affection, and someone you pay to do it. What does it say about a society where we're paying working women to rent their womb for hire?' He goes on and talks about surrogacy being a form of prostitution, a way for the rich to exploit poor women.

I call my husband and tell him about Litz, Rifkin, and the creepy guy with the bird. I am wondering why we did not research the entire landscape of surrogacy before we signed on. My husband asks if it would have mattered, I guess it wouldn't have.

"If you look hard enough you will find a 'coalition against anything,'" he assures me.

But maybe that's what I need to do. Maybe I need to research and read about people and coalitions and organizations of people who hate what I am doing, and who therefore hate me. Their hatred is clear and defined, self-righteous and brilliantly simple.

"Many critics of surrogate motherhood contend that it degrades women by converting them into reproductive vessels," writes a journalist in an *LA Times* article entitled, *Surrogacy Ethics: Surrogate Motherhood: A Wrenching Test of Ethics*. "[Surrogate motherhood] threatens to create a 'breeder class' of poor and minority women, bearing babies for the rich. New York author and feminist Phyllis Chesler calls it 'strip-mining the fertility of the poor.'"

The article goes on to quote Angela R. Holder, clinical professor of pediatrics and law at Yale University's School of Medicine who condemns society's focus on genetically related children: "'People want babies to satisfy their selfish needs, as hostages to fortune, to carry on their names,' she said. Holder opposes legalized surrogacy contracts because she believes that they turn babies into commodities 'by promising them and paying for them, like cars.' Rather than engaging in surrogacy to create new life, more couples ought to adopt needy children, she said."

When I read their proclamations, so seething and angry, I find myself envying their steadfastness, their unwavering belief that what they preach is an absolute truth; how wonderful it must be to know, without a tinge of doubt, that you are right. And that the rest of us, shuffling around day after day in an ambivalent fog, are sadly wrong and mislead.

I think back to Sunday school and how comforting it was to believe that bad people went to hell and good people went to heaven; no wonder I slept so deliciously well as a child.

***

There is a website called EverythingSurrogacy.com, which offers an *EverythingSurrogacy Store!* I am not sure whether the exclamation point is part of the store's name, but as I read further the number of exclamation points used in their catalogue is so astounding that I am led to believe that that particular exclamation point was not a typo. There are three items to choose from in the store: the first is a pair of conception socks. Screen printed by hand in the EverythingSurrogacy.com studio, these socks feature a drawing of a sperm rushing toward an egg, along with the words: *Fertile Thoughts*. "Let's face it," the description says, "infertility treatments, AIs and IVFs are not fun. Why not help relieve some of that tension by brightening up the mood a bit with these funny one size fits all conception socks!" I am assured that they will make a great gift because they are a "fun way of saying 'Good Luck!!!'" But, alas, at the bottom of the page I find that they are sold out of the socks: "**SOLD OUT!!!!**" Yes, over 400 hundred pairs of these socks have been sold in the US, Canada, and UK. It seems that I am not so lucky today.

I move on to the next item: a "blueish lavender" T-shirt with a logo of three birds sitting in a nest admiring a hatched heart. These "race and gender neutral" bird T-shirts are "perfect for gay families, surrogacies, adoptions, and even egg and sperm donation families...what better way to show the loving understanding between yourself and those who assisted you in having a child and vice versa!?!" Perhaps this T-shirt was the inspiration for Mr. Melinger bringing a live bird with him to the hospital in Indianapolis; it wasn't an act of lunacy, it was an act of solidarity, of appreciation! The style of the shirt is particularly special, "due to their flattering cut, they can be worn by any non-pregnant man or woman without looking too big." A non-pregnant man...

The third item in the store is the baby pink "Proud New Mom!" T-shirts, "designed not only for traditional new mothers but women who have become moms via adoption and surrogacy as well!!!!" It is recommended that this shirt be worn by someone like me so that I will never have to worry about the maternity staff at the hospital forgetting who I am. It does strike me as strange that EverythingSurrogacy.com assures me that the shirt will arrive in an "unmarked package, preventing anyone from knowing its content" because I thought the intent was to announce to the world that I am a "Proud New Mom!" Not only are these 100%

high quality, one-size-fits all, pre-shrunk cotton T-shirts roomy enough to fit over clothes or a still pregnant belly, but "after the birth you can take the shirt off and use it as a blanket to help your new baby become accustomed to your scent and bond more easily to you."

An understanding friend, a therapist, a blanket to help you bond with your newborn child, all of this and more for only $15, which includes shipping!

I order one of each.

Good Fences

David McCullough writes in *John Adams*:

On his rounds of Boston as a young lawyer, Adams had often heard a man with a fine voice singing behind the door of an obscure house. One day, curious to know who 'this cheerful mortal' might be, he had knocked at the door, to find a poor shoemaker with a large family living in a single room. Did he find it hard getting by, Adams had asked. 'Sometimes,' the man said. Adams had ordered a pair of shoes. 'I had scarcely got out the door before he began to sing again like a nightingale,' Adams remembered. 'Which was the greatest philosopher? Epictetus, the Greek Stoic philosopher or this shoemaker?' he would ask when telling the story. Epictetus, the Greek Stoic philosopher, had said, among other things, 'It is the difficulties that show what great men are.'

November 1st: Norah feels the baby move for the first time. She calls to tell me the news after I have put my daughter to bed. She tells me she was resting on the couch and suddenly she felt a kick. I remember that I was 18 weeks pregnant with my daughter before I felt her move; Norah is only 14 weeks. As I listen to her describe the fluttering movement she felt, I feel myself let go. I feel myself slip into this glorious moment, leaving my brain and the outside world behind. There is a stirring in my belly, of excitement, of anticipation, of love for this baby who is now about the size of a fist. I clinch my hand and stare at it as Norah talks.

"Good fences make good neighbors." I don't know what Robert Frost would say about co-existing peaceably in New York City apartments; he would probably say, *Move to a farm in Vermont and raise goats.* The main difference between living in an apartment building and living in a house within a neighborhood is space — not living space, but the literal space that separates you and yours from your neighbors. I had no idea just how important this space was until I moved into an apartment. There are five units located on our floor, five different families live in these five units, there is one narrow hallway connecting the apartments, and one small trash room. Needless to say I have been spotted in my pajamas taking the trash out by each man, woman, child and dog who lives on our floor. The space I long for, the space I miss, be it a lawn or a driveway or a sidewalk, allows neighbors freedom, freedom to communicate with each other, or the freedom not to. It is perfectly acceptable in a neighborhood setting to simply wave to your neighbor as you are lugging the groceries out of your car, or taking the trash out, or sitting on the porch reading the paper; and it is equally acceptable to pretend that you don't even see your neighbor, as busy as you are with the groceries, the trash, and the reading: it is called ignoring the polite way. But in an apartment building there is no possible way to ignore politely, not when your neighbor is standing inches away from your face. Of course people do ignore the old fashioned way, but it is not in my genetic make-up to do so.

So I run into my neighbor in the hallway. We chat. The topic of summer comes up and she comments that she never saw us over the summer — were we traveling? I pause, staring at this woman whom I do not know very well, though she seems nice, and she is a mother after all, I decide to do something impulsive and tell her about Norah. This is the first time I have told someone outside of my circle; I feel my heart pounding against my chest as I explain the situation. She listens intently, she nods, raises her eyebrows in surprise, and crosses her arms in front of her. I take a deep breath — it wasn't so bad, really. But before she even has a chance to comment on my unexpected confession, I instinctively know that I have made a grave mistake. The panic of vulnerability, the panic of having just committed an irreversible deed rushes through my body; I feel my face flush red, my hands begin to sweat. And yes, there it is: something has changed in her demeanor, there has been a shift between us that feels oddly like a transfer of power. She proceeds to tell me of a woman whom she knew in California who used the services of a surrogate so that she did not have to gain weight. She then questions me, skeptically, accusingly. *How did you find this surrogate? Aren't you nervous that this woman has complete control over your unborn child? Can you trust her not to smoke or drink or, God forbid, do drugs?*

The more obedient and sincere I am in answering her, the more suspicious and hard-nosed her inquiries become; I think she mistakes my easygoing attitude for naiveté.

"What's wrong with you, anyway?" She asks.

I stare at her, not understanding the question. Am I being rude? Perhaps my face has turned an alarming shade of purple and she's worried. I am trying to think of what to say when she follows up the question with:

"Your body — what's wrong with your body? Why could you carry your daughter?"

She is like a drill sergeant, demanding quick, precise answers, and I give them to her because I don't know what else to do.

"This can't be cheap. How much are you paying her?"

"Enough," I reply.

I resort to throwing out Joan Lunden's name, as if this will give me some legitimacy; and, not surprisingly, it does. Hearing that I have used the same agency as a celebrity lightens the air between us for a moment. The conversation comes full circle with the weight issue again.

"How much did you gain with your daughter?"

And she ends the conversation with one last remark about how lucky I am that I don't have to deal with maternity clothes.

I have this terrible feeling that the issue of weight — of actually not having to gain it in order to attain the prize of one's own biological child — will not play in my favor. This, I did not anticipate. I tell a friend about the conversation with my neighbor.

"Is the bitch overweight?" My friend asks.

"No, not at all," I tell her. "In fact, the bitch is very thin."

Then my friend tells me something I don't want to hear: this is only the beginning.

"Pregnancy, motherhood, children, there's not a more competitive or cut-throat field in the world. People are going to look at you and think you took the easy road — they don't give a damn about your placenta or your uterus or that you almost died in childbirth, they care about the size of your jeans and why and how you can still wear a 4."

"Will it help placate these 'people' if I tell them I would have gladly gained 30 pounds again to carry another baby?" I ask.

"No," my friend says. "Because they won't believe you."

"I feel like I'm in eighth grade again," I say.

"You never left."

When I return home and search for *Identity: Youth and Crisis*, I cannot find it anywhere. My daughter wants to know what I'm looking for. Nothing, I tell her. But she is insistent and knows when I am lying. I am hesitant to tell her because I had hoped she had forgotten about "Mommy's book" and moved onto more interesting things, like her father's *Sports Illustrated*. She tells me she wants to help me and I cannot resist her. So I tell her I'm looking for that book.

"You know, the one that mommy writes in, the one you like to read, too."

She nods her head in excitement and takes my hand and leads me into her room, where I watch her crawl onto her stomach and reach under her bed and retrieve Erikson's book, which she places in my hands.

***

Life keeps moving. Days pass, weeks pass. I make my daughter breakfast in the mornings, we walk to school. I race home to use the three precious hours that I am alone to write, and I try to forget about the question my neighbor asked me: what's wrong with you? I remember as she asked the question how her eyes squinted — out of suspicion? Out of curiosity? Out of her desire for drama? Perhaps all of the above. What I am sure of is how she could never know how many times I have asked the same question of myself, not out of curiosity or suspicion, but out of repulsion and shame. I know what placenta accreta is now, but I had no idea what it was the night I gave birth to my daughter. "Placenta accreta is an abnormally firm attachment of the placenta to the uterine wall," explains an article in *Midwifery Today*.

> Accreta is a potentially fatal complication for the mother due to hemorrhage as blood loss typically ranges from 3000 mls to 5000 mls. Other potentially fatal complications include Disseminating Intravascular Coagulation (DIC), which can result in death or amputation of lower limbs; transfusion reactions, other complications accompanying blood transfusions such as HIV or hepatitis, allo-immunization, fluid overload, and less commonly, infection and multiple organ failure. Surgical morbidity includes: emergency hysterectomy, bowel injury, urological injuries including urethral trauma and bladder lacerations requiring surgical resection. Patients with accreta are at increased risk for blood clots (for example pulmonary embolism) and Adult Respiratory Distress Syndrome...10% of women with placenta accreta die of its complications.

In the article the cause for placenta accreta points to multiple Cesarean sections, along with the rise of elective and non-elective Cesarean sections performed every year. In 2004, cesareans accounted for 29% of all births nationwide; the risk of accreta jumps 40% in women who have had more than one C-section. "Statistics indicate that placenta accreta was a rare occurrence from 1930-1950 — approximately one case in over 30,000 deliveries. From 1950 to 1960, the number increased to one in 19,000 and by 1980 one in 7,000. The most recent information suggests that the incidence has now risen to one in 2,500 deliveries."

But I did not have a Cesarean section with my daughter. There is no convenient reason as to why my placenta stayed put. Perhaps the miscarriage of twins, before I got pregnant with my daughter, and the subsequent DNC performed left scarring on my uterine wall that contributed to the accreta; or maybe it was my daughter's twin whose death at 9 weeks caused complications, and there was nothing to do but wait and let the sac and its contents pass into the toilet; or maybe it was the irregular shape of my uterus, which my doctor discovered the night of my daughter's birth.

Maybe. Perhaps. Possibly. There is no answer, and there never will be an answer to why my body failed to get it right. And I feel at this moment that I am hovering close to that unbearable state of self-pity — oh, this is the danger of *The Memoir* that I fear, its love of drama, the trap of its opened arms calling to me to let it all out, come on now, have a good cry and feel sorry for yourself, life *has* been so unfair to you, hasn't it? And I inch closer to the arms because they are reaching for me, promising safety and understanding; I inch closer, my mouth open, ready to explain how I feel so disgusted with myself not because I cannot become pregnant again, because I can, but because I wasn't good at it. Did I honestly believe that paying another human being — not to paint my house or repair my car — but to do what I could not do: carry a child, the most basic of all human biological functions, would not be complicated? I daresay, I did.

I tuck my daughter into bed; she wants me to tell her about Bad Shark. She has recently discovered sharks, and this discovery has aligned perfectly with her sudden interest in all things dangerous and scary. So I make up a story about Bad Shark who lives in a cave and has no friends because he insists on eating his friends, and now all the mermaids and sea creatures in the ocean have gotten savvy about Bad Shark and will no longer play with him. *Oh, but let's make him Nice Shark now*, my daughter says. So I make him kind, and the mermaids and sea creatures swim to his cave to give him another chance and all is peaceful again. *No, no, no make him Bad Shark now, have him eat everyone*, she insists. And tragically the friends are lured to his cave once again only to become lunch.

It goes on like this for another ten minutes or so: bad shark, nice shark, bad shark. I can see in her eyes the delight in exploring these new emotions of fear and trust, of betrayal and forgiveness, of wielding power over the outcome of a story. But it is getting late and Bad Shark must go back to his cave and rest, he is exhausted, understandably.

I go back to my office to write, and I find the arms are still there, still open, still reaching out for me; and I am tempted — who doesn't want a hand rubbed on the back? A sympathetic tear shed? But I have been there before, I have succumbed to those alluring arms, and each time found its solace fleeting, its intentions indulgent and ultimately unstable, like Bad Shark. I don't want to feel sorry for myself, I simply want to tell my story.

Love Songs

In the eyes of the Catholic Church, our daughter is a bastard. Technically my husband and I are not even married. He is a Catholic; I am not. I wanted a wedding ceremony outside under the trees; his Catholic priest refused to bless a ceremony without the church altar. So we were married outside on a hot, July day in Virginia under two-hundred-year-old sycamore trees. Reverend Knox, a nice Methodist minister, officiated. His sermon was short and sweet, and the only part of it I remember nine years later is this: "Be nice to each other." Be nice to each other. It was the way he said it, the ceremonial tone was suddenly gone, and before our eyes he seemed more like a coach telling his team: the hell with it! Just go and have a good time. And we took his advice.

The real reason why we got married had less to do with love than with being able to sleep in the same bed on family vacations. Sharing a life together was something we had decided years earlier. We have known each other since the seventh grade, we dated through high school, college, and graduate school. For us, marriage was exciting but it was also a technicality, a next step in an organically evolving relationship, very much like our daughter learning to walk and talk; it was inevitable, welcomed, celebrated, but not surprising. The surprise had already occurred, ten years earlier at the age of fifteen when I simply knew I would be with him for the rest of my life. Certainly hormones, the smell of his t-shirts (Speedstick deodorant and sweat) and endless kissing romanticized my realization; but then again, I was a serious teenager, a witness to crumbling marriages and infidelities. My parents had run with a fast crowd when I was growing up (at age nine, I knew what a jigger was and how to use it. I could mix Bloody Marys, Vodka Tonics and my father's favorite, Old Fashions: a jigger of bourbon whiskey, a dash of bitters, a splash of water, a lot of sugar—my father liked extra sugar—one maraschino cherry, one slice of orange, stir and serve on ice), there was little I had not seen.

It is June 19, 1986, a boy's parents are out of town (Chris Savage is his name, he will be dead in five years, a motorcycle accident) and like all teenagers we are desperate for a place of our own, even if only for a few hours. My future husband and I lie together on a twin bed. Voices call from downstairs, beer has been found in the garage, cheering ensues. We lie side by side staring at the ceiling. He is oddly quiet and I just want to make-out, but he hasn't made a move, so I wait. Minutes go by, we have not spoken, he is so still. I am getting bored. I sit up, leaning on my arm, and stare at him. What I see is something I am not prepared for, he is crying. I have never seen a sixteen-year-old boy cry before. I have seen dozens of sixteen-year-old girls cry and it is nothing like this. Girls are loud, violent, their faces turn different shades of red and purple, limbs flail, snot and tears smear the face like war paint, words are inaudible. His face is not red, his breathing is calm, only his hands shake slightly; he suddenly looks old to me. He is crying because Len Bias is dead. The twenty-two-year-old University of Maryland basketball player was found dead from a cocaine overdose, just forty-eight hours after being drafted by the Boston Celtics. I am only fifteen and I don't understand why he is so upset over the death of someone whom he didn't know. He admired Len Bias as a basketball player, I get that, but he didn't know him personally. I say nothing. I pat him on the hand like I have seen older people do. Then suddenly he pulls me to him and holds me close, he holds me tightly and there is nothing sexual or erotic about this embrace; it is the first time in my life that I feel the clinch of hands and arms seeking safety and comfort in me. The voices of our friends downstairs, the sound of my heart beating, his breathing, all are silenced by something in this room that suddenly feels broken. I move to stand up, I do not have the patience or the courage to endure this, this unhappiness over a dead athlete, but he resists my movement and holds on tighter, and at some point my spine relaxes, my body gives in to his, the stubborn immaturity of me retracts. He has brought me here, to this grief, to this loneliness, to this knot of complexities, and it is almost unbearable, but for the warmth of his hand on the back of my neck.

This wondrous boy has given me a glimpse of an entire life and how to survive it; but of course I don't know this yet.

***

> *'I'm going to marry you whether you like it or not.'*
> He took her face into his hands and looked longingly at her mouth. *'I'm going to marry you till you puke.'*

I have always loved this marriage proposal in Lorrie Moore's short story, "Terrific Mother." Martin proposes to Adrienne during a terrible time in her life; she is depressed and cannot believe he could really love her, much less want to marry her. It is possibly the least romantic marriage proposal in history, though to me it is the most endearing. It wipes away the schmaltz, the drama, it debunks the myths, the lies, it skips over the white dress, the seated dinner for two-hundred, the honeymoon suite, the coveted Herend place setting, and goes straight to the morning after, to the head resting on the toilet, the hair matted with last night's chicken, the soiled clothes balled up in a corner, and to the apologies uttered while hands rub a back and kiss a shoulder, despite the stench.

When you are young and in love (and I mean really young, as in you may or may not have a driver's license yet, or you may even still use a pacifier) the outside world literally does not matter, in some ways it does not exist. Already egocentric by nature, young love is self-absorbed, arrogant, narcissistic, indulgent; and it is arguably the last time in life when two people are untouchable, protected, wholly oblivious to judgment, social pressures, opinions. I had forgotten about that world until today, when my daughter had a play-date with a boy from her class. We meet the boy and his mother at Alice's Tea Cup, a small café that serves tea and scones. Since September the two have been inseparable at school; I have watched them together on days when I volunteer at the library. Their teacher has told me how fond they are of each other, and this fondness is apparent in the mornings during drop-off and in the afternoons during pick-up as they stand together in line giggling. The boy is five, two years older than my daughter, with kind blue eyes and an undeniable sweetness beneath his boyish energy. His mother informs me that he has never asked for a play-date with a girl before.

I allow my daughter to wear whatever she likes. I sit on her floor and watch as she stands at the closet with her arms crossed, assessing her choices. She picks out a light blue, short sleeve corduroy dress with a round collar; beneath it she will wear a long-sleeve white T-shirt with tulle around the cuffs; and as for tights, a pair of orange, red, green and blue striped. And though she would like to wear her yellow-sequined sling-back heels, she settles for the knee-high brown boots embroidered with pink and purple flowers. She will carry a purple and white purse containing a plastic cell phone, her beloved pacifier and her lovey, a small, yellow wash cloth that she has named "Peeta." We skip to the café.

We order tea, pumpkin scones with clotted cream and strawberry jam, homemade graham crackers and honey. With these two children there is no "warm-up," no time needed to get comfortable with each other, they are at once giggling, sitting side-by-side in the booth, wrestling. She is too busy flirting to eat; he is trying to eat in between the giggling and full body hugs my daughter bestows upon him. The boy's mother and I watch, you cannot help but watch. My daughter pulls her pacifier from her purse and shows it to her friend, she is gushing with pride; he smiles, clearly unimpressed (he is almost six, after all), but he is so smitten with her that he cannot help but see its charm. For a split second their bodies are still as they stare into each other's eyes — but this stillness proves too much and in an instant my daughter is on top of him again, her arms around his neck, her toothy grin an inch away from his face as his hand pats her back gently. Then he excuses himself from the table to use the bathroom and my daughter lies down in the booth with her legs in the air, her dress folds over her head exposing her falling tights, her belly button and her bottom, which is wet because she has peed. I try to get her to sit up (I didn't bring an extra set of clothes) as her friend heads back to the table, but she refuses — she refuses because she doesn't care. *He will love me, wet bum, nasty pacifier, ragged little wash cloth and all!* The boy sits down next to her and now my daughter is hugging him again, kissing his face, repeating to him: *I love you! I love you so much! I love you!* He only smiles, offering himself up to her and her silly antics of love and tackling. People begin to stare. The waitresses stare, the busboy stares, the chef even comes out for a look. Some smile, some are stunned, but the lure of these two children is undeniable because what we are witnessing is an overture, a preface, an introduction to love; for these two the real thing will not come for years, but for the rest of us who know love in its maturity, in its various forms of shame, fear, hurt, and disappointment, theirs is a reminder of that sweet time, right before the story begins.

***

I have been downloading love songs onto my daughter's I-Pod. This I-Pod was a gift from her godfather on her second birthday. Her godfather is a New York City bachelor who lives in Tribeca and owns a massage table and a 100-inch screen TV and goes to spas in places like Mexico to cleanse his body and mind. In the course of this downloading I have not forgotten about her musical taste (it is her I-Pod after all), downloaded is the soundtrack from her beloved Mary Poppins, all of Dan Zanes, and The Best of Johnny Cash. When my husband and I were dating I used to make him mixed tapes, love letters in the form of songs that I would spend hours preparing. No matter who you are, no matter how evolved your taste, I dare anyone to deny their participation in the adolescent pastime of making mixes for their mates. Not only were the songs themselves important but the sequencing of the songs was equally vital. The tape would always begin with something catchy, like Van Morrison's, "Brown-Eyed Girl," The Beach Boys' "Wouldn't It Be Nice," or America's "Sister Golden Hair;" and then somewhere in the middle of the tape the theme would change, the guitar riffs would become edgier as the tone of the mix shifted to the darker side of love. Fleetwood Mac's "Go Your Own Way," Dire Straits, "Romeo and Juliet," Aerosmith's, "Cryin'," The Eagles, "Wasted Time;" all of these clichéd sentiments blasted from the tape like a snarl, like a warning. I was always drawn to this part of the mix, when love goes terribly wrong, when the good times are only memories, and love is forever transformed into a dichotomous state of bitterness and remorse, triumph and defeat, retribution and apologies.

At the moment I am listening to duets, and I keep going back to the same song: Neil Diamond and Barbra Streisand's, "You Don't Bring Me Flowers." At the beginning of the song when Neil's smooth, deep voice breaks in: "You hardly talk to me anymore, when I come through the door at the end of the day," I rest my head on my desk and wish I had a fainting couch. This kind of heartbreak is addictive, like Gummy Bears. There is something beautiful about the pain in their voices, about this loss of love channeled through clichés and tired metaphors. After listening to dozens of more love songs I realize that what makes a good love song are those clichés and metaphors; the clever songs don't work. Take Lyle Lovett's, "Nobody Knows Me," that begins, "I like cream in my coffee and I like to sleep late on Sundays..." Though his voice is undeniably gorgeous and the hurt is there, it's there, man! He's already lost me before the second verse. He's making me work too hard for this heartbreak, and I don't want to work for it, I don't want to draw my own conclusions from the cream in the coffee, I don't want poetry. I want to lie on that fainting couch (wherever that may be) and be spoon-fed pain, anguish, despair, via small words and short sentences. I want to hear Journey's Steve Perry belt out: "When I'm alone, all by myself, you're out with someone else, lovin', touchin', squeezin' each other;" I want to hear Neil sing again about those "used to bes [that] don't count anymore, they just lay on the floor 'til we sweep them away." Because if I listen to these songs enough times I can even push out a few tears for them, but mostly for myself.

"How does marriage change things?" the question that has been directed at me many times over these past ten years, which I have never had an answer for, finally comes to me: You no longer make loves mixes for your mate, you make them for yourself. Listening to love songs is pure indulgence, it is self-absorption, it is self-pity for self-pity's sake that can be replayed over and over again to your heart's content, void of witnesses, explanations, solutions. In theory, I shouldn't be moved by

Journey's song about "a small town girl living in a lonely world, [who] took the midnight train going anywhere," but I am. Such songs cry out for late-night drives alone with one's heartbreak and disappointment—who hasn't taken such a drive? And when the time comes to return home, who hasn't sat in their car, in the cold silence, realizing nothing has been solved, and yet somehow feeling better?

In marriage there is a constant tendency towards resolution, a panic to solve problems quickly so that time spent in that cloudy state of confusion, of anger and fear, can be minimized, or better yet, avoided completely. A clouded mind is dangerous, it lacks judgment, it voices cruel opinions, it is careless. The institution of marriage works best when life, within its walls, is black and white. The role of good guy and bad guy shifts back and forth, like a friendly game of catch, offences happen, the guilty party steps forward, amends are made, and a good night sleep is had by all. Safety at any cost, that seems to be marriage's aim. But what happens when there is no good guy or bad guy, when the offense is something intangible or perhaps not even an offense at all? What happens when there is no clear-cut resolution?

Tomorrow I go in for my annual "placenta check-up." I will lie inside the capsule of an MRI machine, with foam in my ears, for anywhere from thirty to forty minutes, while a technician takes pictures of this strange nodule attached to my uterine wall. My doctors have been monitoring this piece of placenta for three years now with nothing remarkable to report other than it appears to be shrinking and has left in its wake a mess of things in my uterus. I have my suspicions that somewhere in some obscure medical journal I am Patient A, the white female still carrying placenta around three years after giving birth. I do not tell my husband about my appointment tomorrow. The topic of my placenta need not inhabit our conversation or bed tonight; and only after we turn out the lights does this decision worry me. This is not like me, I leave nothing to the imagination when it comes to us. The obvious repercussions of what this piece of placenta has done to our family have been discussed, argued, dragged, kicked, and kicked again, mostly by me. Many times over I have forced him to see that because of me we can never have another child a normal way; because of me he is faced with the same intrusive questions, the same tiresome explanations; because of me the outside world that we successfully shut out when we were young has now been let in to view our private struggle. Because of me we will be the subject of cocktail chatter among acquaintances, or worse, complete strangers. Because of me people will study our second child, looking for genetic resemblances, they will ask questions about my placenta as if my body were a recipe for a complicated cheesecake; and yes, we will be "That couple," or "That friend," our child, "That child who was born from a surrogate."

"How can I say this gently?" my friend from San Diego asks me over the phone one evening. "People really don't care about your situation."

"But don't you see?" I explain. "That is exactly my point, people who do not care about me or my family have been given open access to us, to judge, to question, to pry. To shut them out is a disservice to Norah, and yet to let them in is physically painful for me. Do you see my predicament?" Yes, she does, and she understands it all too well. She has been known to feign deafness at cocktail parties when personal questions are directed at her; it is a rare talent that I envy.

My husband, on the other hand, feels completely different than me.

"None of that matters," is his response to all of it. "Who cares what anyone thinks."

As we lie in the darkness an infamous figure from our past by the name of Mary Kelley comes to my mind. She is an old friend of my mother's, a woman from the old school who never wore pants, arrived at all parties at exactly the time given on the invitation, and delivered the one-liners she was famous for with the coolness and determination of an assassin: "You look so tired all the time," "Have you put on weight?" "I see you're still drinking." On the day of our wedding my husband and I stood in a receiving line (because that is what my mother told us to do) and greeted our 300 guests, one by one. Somewhere in the middle of that endless line of well-wishers, Mary Kelley stood before us in her knee-length summer suit, not smiling (she never smiled), but examining closely. Then she turned her back to me, looked at my husband and said, "You are the catch of the century."

I turn and look at my husband in the shadowed darkness of our room. What do you say to the catch of the century when you know he is right? When I ask him this question he breaks into a smile, that heartbreaking smile that made little old ladies, even the likes of Mary Kelley, swoon.

I am madly in love with this man, whom I was clever enough to marry, but I am also stuck in a conflict between practicality and something that feels primal, steeped in the folds of my biology, isolated by the features of maternal instincts of which a man has no possession or real understanding, not because he is imperceptive, but because he isn't wired to understand it. I have been stuck for months now and my husband has said all the right things that, in theory, should have resolved the confusion and sadness and brought me back, the old me. But what he cannot understand right now is how much this sadness, this clouding of the mind has taken hold, like hunger or thirst, and is beyond my control, but evidently necessary in my search for resolution. I need Steve Perry and Neil Diamond precisely because they cannot give me a solution, just wonderfully corny music.

Night Swimming

It is only when I leave New York City that I am reminded of its intensity. When you live here you feel it walking down the street, you hear it in voices, car horns, ambulance sirens, barking dogs, the incessant beeping of trucks that seem to be in a perpetual state of reverse. You feel it, but over time this intensity becomes a part of you, like callused feet, and you adapt. And one day you find your pace has sped up, street noises are dulled, your patience has transformed from quiet waiting to foot tapping and heavy breathing, and you forget to say hello to strangers for no other reason than you're walking too fast.

When I step off the plane in Indianapolis I speed-walk through the airport, speed-dial my husband at work, stop to buy a bottle of water, speed-dial Norah who waits for me outside of baggage claim, then a quick stop at the bathroom where I speed-dial my babysitter to check on my daughter. I am at the airport exit before half the people on my flight have even deplaned. As I walk out the door I hear a voice calling, *Excuse me! Excuse me!* I turn and a woman is hurrying toward me, carrying the scarf I had dropped somewhere along the way.

Norah's doctor recommended an amniocentesis, as did mine, because of my geriatric age of 35. I find the exact definition for an amniocentesis in a medical encyclopedia: *a diagnostic procedure performed by inserting a hollow needle through the abdominal wall into the uterus and withdrawing a small amount of fluid from the sac surrounding the fetus.* The test is performed in order to detect chromosomal disorders and other rare, inherited metabolic disorders. I knew this definition in general terms, but lately I find myself seeking out reference books and dictionaries for exact definitions and explanations. Perhaps the act of actually holding a book in my hand and reading a neatly typed scientific meaning, somehow gives me a sense of control, or maybe it isn't control but the sense that somebody out there has these terms under control, and thus they seem less daunting to me. Norah has never had an amniocentesis, and she is nervous. I am not doing so well myself, anxiety has been milling around the pit of my stomach since early October when the appointment was made. I am not worried about the results of the amnio, I know the baby is fine just as I knew my daughter was fine when I had the amnio with her. I have no explanation to why this is but it is the same sixth sense that wakes me up at night seconds before my daughter calls to me. I am worried because it is not my belly that will be penetrated by the needle, it is not my doctor, one of the best in New York City, performing the procedure, it is not my body that will go straight home and obediently lie in bed for five days, it is Norah's. I speak with my doctor and she reiterates what I already know, what I remember well: after the amnio Norah must rest, no work, no play, no vacuuming, no heavy lifting, no baths, no flying for a week.

Norah has spoken to the coordinator at the hospital in Indianapolis about the amnio, and she no longer feels nervous about the procedure. I called this same coordinator to inquire about their patient protocol for amnios and she successfully sent me into a full-blown panic. She was very nice, cheerful actually, and quick to giggle. I was not quick to giggle and I began to sweat within minutes of our conversation.

"How many days rest do you recommend after the amnio?" I asked. She giggled.

"Days? Oh no, we don't recommend days of rest, you should just take it easy for the rest of the day, you can even drive yourself home if you want to."

I explained to her that it was not me who would be having the amnio, but Norah, my surrogate.

"You're *what*?" she asked.

I lay down on the kitchen floor.

"You're not Norah?" She was confused. I listened to pages being turned and shuffled rapidly, her breathing had grown uneasy. I explained to her my situation, then there was a long, awkward pause; she didn't know what to say.

"What about no heavy lifting and no baths?" I asked.

"Well, I think if you want to take a bath it's all right, but I expect heavy lifting isn't a good idea anyway."

I thanked her for her time and hung up the phone.

I trust Norah. I would not have signed the contract with her back in April if I didn't inherently know that I could trust her. What I am experiencing now in our story is a shift, a plot twist so to speak, that has nothing to do with trust. Trust is easy, trust is palpable in Norah's voice, in her glowing skin; trust wraps its arms around me when I watch programs about babies born to smokers, drinkers, and drug-addicts; trust empties my head and helps me sleep at night. What keeps me awake now is control, more specifically, my lack of it. When I went through IVF over the summer and Norah gave herself shots that depended on her uterus being ready for our embryos, I never worried; after she was pregnant and she continued to give herself progesterone shots in the bum, I never worried, I never wondered whether or not she was doing them correctly or doing them exactly every 24-hours. But this amnio is different, it feels different because the baby is no longer a concept, a statistic, a positive reading on a pregnancy test. I study old ultrasound pictures of my daughter at 19 weeks, at her small, round head, the turned-up nose, at her hands and fingers so delicate, almost translucent, as if they might disintegrate into the black and white fuzz like dust. When I began to leak amniotic fluid at 32 weeks with my daughter, when the contractions began, when Dr. Edelman looked me in the eye and said, "You are going to deliver this baby today," and even after I was given shots of prenatal steroids to pump up my daughter's lungs, I knew, without a doubt, that I could stop labor. After 24-hours, when the contractions had stopped and my daughter's heart rate calmed to a steady pace, my doctors checked me into the hospital and told me to try and lie on my left side, this might help keep the baby stable, they said. For five weeks I lay on the hospital bed on my left side, all day and all night, while eating, while sleeping, while reading; when I used the toilet I balanced on my left butt cheek. At the age of nine I enforced the seatbelt law on anyone who rode in our car; in 1979 there was no seatbelt law in the state of Virginia, that would come nine years later. But it is a comforting place, isn't it? Protected by rules, guarantees, statistics, the illusion of control transforms into something as tangible as a hand on a back guiding you, promising somewhere safe. It is difficult to push the hand away, even when you allow yourself to see that it was never there in the first place.

I can ask Norah to please rest, I can drive her home from the hospital and tuck her in bed with magazines and bottles of water, place flowers on her bedside table and order dinner in for her family, but when I walk out of her home and get in a taxi and head for the airport, I can do nothing but hope she will do the right thing.

I watch Norah get out of her car and walk to me, her arms outstretched. As we embrace I feel my body relax, my heart rate slows down; she is a person blessed with a calm aura, she is never in a hurry. In August, on the day of the transfer when the doctor inserted our embryos into Norah, the nurse gave her strict instructions to *lie*, not sit, in bed for the next twenty-four hours. On the way back to the hotel, on Interstate 495, we got a flat tire. Cars, trucks, eighteen-wheelers charged past us, shaking our car; minutes later it began to rain. There was no median, and therefore no room, to change the tire safely. It was four o'clock, Washington DC rush hour had just begun. While my husband called his brother and AAA and read through the chapter in the owner's manual on changing tires, I looked deep within myself to find the strength to not have a nervous break down. Norah sat in the backseat, calm and relaxed. *I can change a flat tire, you know*, she said. I tried to smile. *Ashley, don't worry, the embryos are not going to fall out*, she added. Eventually my brother-in-law came to the rescue and picked Norah and me up, delivering her safely to her hotel, while my husband stayed behind with the flat-tire and the owner's manual and waited for AAA.

And Norah was right, the embryos didn't fall out.

On the drive to the hospital conversation is easy, effortless. I ask her if she is nervous about the amnio, she says she is not and I believe her. During the long drive there are no awkward pauses, it's as if we're old friends. And we are friends, our friendship is real, if I had met Norah under different circumstances we would have hit it off immediately. She is smart, open, approachable, funny—she is a friend you would not hesitate to call at three in the morning if you needed her, which adds to the torment I feel in not disclosing to her how utterly lost I feel, not as her friend, but as the "Intended Mother." Here again is another dichotomy to balance: a friendship between two women, and a legal partnership between a surrogate and an intended mother. Each role bears a different responsibility, a different obligation, expectations and emotions shift depending on the circumstance. Riding in the car next to her, I cannot tell if she is showing because she is wearing a winter coat, and for a few minutes I forget that she is my surrogate, she is simply my friend, pointing out landmarks, talking about her kids, and her love of photography. As Norah talks I look out the window at the corn fields, the farm houses, the flat land that stretches beyond the horizon; there is so much empty space, so much silence. We haven't seen another car in the last few miles, much less a human being. I roll down my window and smell cold air, damp soil, manure. I see cows, horses, goats, the occasional dog, over there a tractor, a silo. I am in a John Cougar Mellencamp music video with all of its tributes and salutes to Americana. For a moment I have to remind myself why I am here, but the conversation must inevitably shift back to the baby, to how Norah is feeling, sleeping, is she craving anything interesting? She says she is a little tired and the baby never stops moving. I smile, nod my head like I understand, but what I feel is a pit in my stomach, a tightening in the throat that perhaps hints at self-pity, or is it something more primal, hormonal, as I sit just inches away from my 17-week-old fetus, separated only by another woman's body, a woman who happens to also be my friend?

Never do business with friends, an adage my father reiterated to me over the years, it complicates things even in the most ideal situations. As usual, he is right.

The hospital is magnificent. It looks like a university campus or a large shopping mall. Not only will Norah deliver here, but her doctor's office is located here, as well as a hotel, located only one floor up from labor and delivery. We are greeted by a social worker. She is a small, blonde-haired woman, early fifties,

I guess. Her name is Pam. It says so on a tag pinned to her blue blazer; she holds a clipboard, and a pager is attached to her belt. She immediately hugs me and congratulates me. I look around, it is so quiet, there are no nurses scurrying around, no crying babies, no pregnant women walking up and down the hallway in hospital gowns, just wide empty corridors and mauve wall-to-wall industrial carpeting; I feel like I'm in rehab.

Pam presses her hand gently against my back as she gives me a tour of the labor and delivery wing which has been renovated. Norah has delivered here before so she sits out for this. The rooms are large, with floor-to-ceiling windows, custom cabinetry, a lot of glass and sparkling chrome, there are soft arm chairs and small couches and televisions, the color scheme is also mauve.

"Sometimes we have eight to ten people in here to watch the birth," Pam says. The hospital beds and monitoring equipment sit like thrones in the middle of the room, bowls of lollipops have been placed on all bed-side tables.

"Everyone loves lollipops," she tells me.

I ask her if it is always this quiet and she nods proudly. We walk past a room, the door is closed, I can hear voices, but only slightly.

"This mommy came in earlier this morning, I think she's about to have the baby," Pam whispers.

When I was in labor with my daughter at New York Presbyterian Hospital, a fully-dressed woman, hunched over, appeared in the doorway of my room yelling, *Where the hell is my room? It's coming! It's coming!* She stood in the doorway bent over with her hands gripping her knees, her dark, tangled hair covering her face, she looked like Alice Cooper. Our eyes locked, and in that spilt second she revealed to me a terrible secret of motherhood: *you're all alone in this, no matter what they tell you.* Then her husband appeared, nervous and small, carrying a suitcase. He escorted her out of the room and she mumbled something about missing the end of *Jeopardy* as they disappeared.

We walk down the hall to the nursery and find that it is empty.

"This is normal," Pam tells me. "Nowadays all the mothers want the babies in their rooms with them."

The empty plastic bassinets are lined up side-by-side in front of the window, like seats in a stadium. There are rocking chairs and plastic bathtubs, there are bottles and jars and tubes of ointment and stacks of tiny diapers on tables. The walls are bordered with teddy bear wallpaper, chubby bears tumbling in clouds of pink and blue; on the side wall hang two prints, one of a stork carrying a baby wrapped in a blue blanket, the other of a stork carrying a baby wrapped in a pink blanket. The babies have round, pink cheeks and dimpled chins and one blonde curl sitting erect on top of their heads. My eyes return to the stork carrying the baby in the pink blanket, the bird is smiling a little too widely, its eyes bulge out of its head, its slanted eyebrows give it a devilish look; it is unclear whether it wants to eat the baby or drop it to its death.

There is a small room adjacent to the nursery, where mothers and fathers can spend time with their babies. Pam tells me to go in. I hesitate.

"Go ahead, take a seat in the rocker, try it out."

I walk into the room. I've never actually been in a room like this. With my daughter I was bed-ridden, she was always brought to me. I am afraid to touch anything because I haven't washed my hands. Pam stands in the doorway, her clipboard pressed to her chest, smiling; then her beeper goes off, and she holds her finger up to me and disappears. I am left standing alone in this room with no windows, it smells of a strong cleanser with a hint of baby shampoo. I sit down in the rocking chair, it lurches backwards, the front feet of the chair lift off the floor and I grab onto the arm rests, pushing against gravity, bringing the chair's feet back down to the floor in a hard slam that seems to echo throughout the entire maternity ward. I sit quietly, I do not move until Pam returns.

Next, I am given a tour of the hotel rooms, just one floor up. The rooms are plain, like those in a Holiday Inn, with small kitchens and queen-sized beds and uncomfortable pull-out couches and large TVs; here, too, the color scheme is mauve. There is a continental breakfast served in the lounge from 7 to 9, free of charge. *All of this for $80,* the hotel manager tells me.

I call my husband from the bathroom.

"Everyone is so nice," I tell him. "It's strange."

He tells me it is not strange, it's the Midwest, enjoy it. Then I feel a surge of air in my chest, and I have to catch my breath as I look around the bathroom, at the empty stalls and fluorescent lights buzzing overhead.

"I don't want to be here," I whisper.

"I know." I listen to his voice, he too is blessed with a calm aura and a happy disposition, plus he is a man, literal thinking comes naturally.

"But you need to get out of the bathroom," he adds.

He is right. But at the moment I cannot move and as I grip the phone to my ear I remember back to one particular night when I was nine and I lay in bed staring at my mother who sat next to me, smoothing her hand across my forehead. *I don't want to grow up*, I said to her. *Oh, you have a long time before then*, she said. But she lied, it wasn't a long time at all, twenty-six years was an instant, a blink of time, and here I am alone in a public restroom on the second floor of a hospital in the middle of Indiana. Hiding.

I understand now why my mother lied, and I am sure that night during my ninth year wasn't the first time. I lie more as a mother than I ever did before. This lying has come about so naturally I often wonder if it is part of our evolutionary process: our young are more likely to be hurt by our own emotions than by predators. So I lie, deceive, or to put it more benignly, I act in order to protect. I leave the bathroom to find Norah standing before me, she has removed her coat and I stare at the round bump below her abdomen. I smile, wrap my arm around hers, and rave about the hospital facilities.

In the waiting room we fill out paper work and once again explain our situation to the confused secretary behind the desk. We are led into a room. Norah undresses and lies down on the table. I look for a place to stand, the room is small and I don't want to be in the way. There is nervous laughter as the ultrasound technician spreads lubricant on Norah's belly that is streaked with stretch marks from five previous pregnancies; I think the marks are beautiful, like intricate tribal tattoos, and the technician agrees, Norah thinks they are hideous and tells us we are crazy. Then I back into the desk, tipping over a tray of papers that crashes to the floor. As I bend down to clean up the mess I feel tears streaming down my face, I turn my back to Norah and the technician and curse myself. The lights shut off and the screen flashes on. I stand up slowly and turn toward the monitor, and there he is: the head, the arms, the legs, the feet, the heart beating, the brain, the kidneys. He is measuring right on track, seventeen weeks, a late April due date is certain. He turns somersaults, exposing his tiny bum to the screen. His movements are quick, elusive, in and out of sight he moves, his skin green in the light then dark as he moves further inside the womb. *Love set you going like a fat, gold watch,* the first line of Sylvia Plath's poem about the birth of her child enters my mind like lyrics to a song; I sing it over and over again in my head as he glides like a swimmer back and forth, his arms floating up over his head, his body twisting, his back now turned. His head peers over his shoulder, as if he knows he is being watched.

"Do you still want to go through with this?" the technician asks.

I am not sure if she is talking to me or to Norah, and at first I think she is referring to my decision to use a surrogate, which strikes me as odd because it's a little late to have second thoughts about that. But as she shuts off the screen I realize what this is.

"The baby looks fine," she adds. "I just wanted to make sure you still wanted the amnio. I assume you read about the risks."

My reaction to her question is a physical one: my shoulders, my head, my arms, my spine, my entire body seems to collapse into itself; it feels like the wind has been knocked out of me. Of course I know the risks, I know what the statistics are, I know that 1 out of every 100 women will miscarry after an amnio, I know there are risks to Norah, a risk of a uterine infection and less serious side effects like cramping and bleeding, of course I know all of this. I sit down and glance at Norah, she stares up at me and smiles.

"Whatever you want to do, Ashley," Norah says. She stares up at the ceiling, she is calm, completely content with whatever decision I make.

I stare at the technician who has now turned away from me and I feel betrayed by her, I thought she was my friend — didn't we share a laugh only moments ago? But I can see that she is not my friend. Superstitions and doubts begin racing through my head: perhaps this is a sign from God, this crazy technician was sent to stop me from going through with the amnio because there will be a mishap, the needle will slip or killer bacteria will find its way into the womb and the baby won't survive it. What other explanation can there be? Everything was going so smoothly, then suddenly this woman decides to voice a warning moments before the procedure? Or maybe I have it all wrong, she was not sent by God but by the devil, tempting me, luring me away from the peace of my decision into a whirling state of confusion. I think of a paper I wrote in high school on *Dr. Faustus,* about the good angel and the bad angel that visit him before he signs his life over to the devil, urging him to do it, urging him not to do it; and how ultimately he makes the wrong decision.

I stand up. The technician sits with her back to me, sorting through the ultrasound pictures. The clearing of her throat, her deep sighs, her hand reaching to pat Norah's, all hint at something self-righteous and smug; her dislike of me and my decisions are clear now. Does she think I have it easy? Does she look at me and think: *Easy for you to stand there while this nice woman takes an 8-inch needle to the abdomen for your child! Must be nice.* But what she could never imagine is how much I understand where she is coming from.

I tell Norah that I have to use the bathroom and I walk out of the room, out of the office, and stand in front of the elevators. I push the elevator button and wait. The elevator doors open and I get in. We are on the 4th floor, so I push 5. The elevator doors close, within a few seconds the doors open to the 5th floor. I wait. Nothing happens, so I push 4. The elevator moves down, the doors open and I step out of the elevator to find myself in the same place where I started; this is what hell must be like.

I walk back into the lobby of the doctor's office and stand in the hallway outside of the examining room. I stare down at the floor, at the mauve carpet. In describing the different life cycles of a human being, Erik H. Erikson writes of the aging person as one "who has taken care of things and people and has adapted himself to the triumphs and disappointments of being, and by necessity,

the originator of others and the generator of things and ideas."
He pinpoints a word that in his opinion best describes an aging
person's state of mind: integrity.

> [Integrity] is the acceptance of one's one and only
> life cycle and of the people who have become
> significant to it as something that had to be and
> that, by necessity, permitted of no substitutions.
> It thus means a new and different love of one's
> parents, free of the wish that they should have
> been different, and an acceptance of the fact
> that one's life is one's own responsibility. It is a
> sense of comradeship with men and women of
> distant times and of different pursuits who have
> created orders and objects and sayings conveying
> human dignity and love. Although aware of the
> relativity of all the various life styles which have
> given meaning to human striving, the possessor
> of integrity is ready to defend the dignity of his
> own life style against all physical and economic
> threats. For he knows that an individual life is
> the accidental coincidence of but one segment
> of history, and that for him all human integrity
> stands and falls with the one style of integrity of
> which he partakes.

I think of the rose garden my mother and grandmother shared.
I remember their tireless devotion to the 125 rose bushes they
kept alive year after year despite beetles and black spot and too
much rain. "Double Delight" was my favorite rose, the rose my
mother would place in a glass and set next to my bed on summer
evenings. It was a rose with a strong, sweet smell, its name
derived from the two colors of it petals, a blood pink and white,
that bled into each other like paint in a watercolor. I can still see its
name carefully written in my grandmother's hand on the square
metal stake that she drove into the ground in front of each rose
bush, like small headstones. I think of how simple life was when
I was that seven-year-old girl hanging on the fence, watching my

mother and grandmother in their wide-brimmed hats work in the garden, how simple it was to be the observer, or rather to believe that I was just the observer, safe from hard work and bloodied hands. Years passed, their work in the rose garden continued as it always had beginning in early spring, unchanged and consistent unlike my body that grew and changed along with my constantly shifting perspective and beliefs. I recall one spring during my teenage years asking my mother what was wrong with getting roses at the florist shop down the street, the upkeep of the garden seemed like an awful lot of trouble. I did not yet understand that dependency and growing up are not separate states of being, but in fact they are shared, from birth they are a partnership, a negotiation back and forth between rules and compromises, circumstances and intent, falling-outs and reconciliations, rest and work. The desire to be needed, and the necessity to care for those who need it, is the life cycle about which Erikson writes, it defines who we are, its continuation the only legacy we have left after those before us die. It is only at this moment, standing alone in the narrow hallway of the doctor's office, thinking of that rose garden that is now buried beneath a housing development, of my mother, and of my grandmother who has been dead for twelve years now, that I understand this. I am here now, the fence is long gone, all I have is what has been lovingly passed on to me. I think of my grandmother sitting across from me, of her straight back and strong shoulders, of her words of survival: *I got moving, that's what I did. That's just what you do.*

I walk back into the room. Both the technician and Norah look at me. I hold Norah's hand and tell her I would like to stick with my original decision.

The doctor enters the room, she is a woman who looks to be my age. She has done her homework on us, there are no awkward questions, explanations are unnecessary. Another woman enters the room and the technician stands up, apparently she is leaving. The technician wishes Norah the best of luck, then she leaves without a word to me. The new woman sits down at the computer and introduces herself, she spreads more jelly onto Norah's abdomen, then places the wand on her stomach. The doctor tells Norah she will feel a pinch, then she inserts three needles into

Norah's abdomen one at a time, and as we watch on the screen the point of the needle penetrate the sac, the baby's movement stops, it is suddenly still. I stare at the hand, the shoulder, the head, suspended in the fluid of the womb like debris, like something fleshy, though lifeless. But as the needle is removed he begins to move again, the arm waving, the legs swimming, still swimming, I imagine, even after the screen turns black.

I take a taxi to the airport. The driver is a woman, an irrelevant detail which I am hesitant to divulge because she gets us lost. But she is a nice woman who made a wrong turn and I appreciate her prudence when we stop at a gas station for directions, and I appreciate her discretion when she does not ask me why I am visiting Indiana or what I do in New York or if I have a family. We drive in circles without conversation.

As the plane takes off from Indianapolis I feel a release, a weight removed. For the next two hours I will be nobody, anonymity is a wonderful thing. It feels like diving to the bottom of a swimming pool and resting there, in silent oblivion.

The Bowl

There was an essay in *The New York Times*, "Modern Love" section last March entitled, "Truly, Madly, Guiltily." I had torn the essay out of the paper and saved it, not knowing that Sunday morning its subject matter would be controversial and that its author, Ayelet Waldman, would appear on *Oprah* to defend it. What moved me about the article happened to be the same topic that caused a great deal of outrage among mothers in America; all of this rage hinging on one line in the essay: "I love my husband more than I love my children." I found this confession fascinating, not because it was radical but because, to me, it was familiar. My mother-in-law has always said there are two kinds of parents: those who put their children and their children's needs before themselves, and those who put themselves and their needs before their children. She and my father-in-law have been happily married 44 years and do love each other dearly, but she does not hesitate to admit that she falls into the category of parents who always put their children's needs first. She believes this is the only way to ensure good, secure children who will then grow up to be good, secure adults. She raised four boys who might be four of the most perfect men on the planet.

In the hospital, the night before my daughter was born, my husband asked me if I would love our daughter more than him. I remember there was a playfulness to his tone, if anything he was a bit embarrassed. The question of love and preference is a high stakes question, it is one that can only be asked in the most trusting of circumstances, and it is usually asked only if you know you will get the answer you are looking for. And like all questions, its context was just as important as the answer: we both had been spoiled with a long history together, we were used to loving each other, solely, now a new person would be added to the team, the dynamics would inevitably be different, love and attention would have to be shared, rationed, measured. So for us his question was pragmatic, sweet, and ultimately necessary. That night in the hospital I thought about this child whom I wanted so desperately, whom I had worked and sacrificed for, and I looked at my husband who smiled shyly and I said, "No. But I will only love you a little bit more." He was satisfied, as was I, and it felt good to have that settled. I did not feel guilty about it, and the idea that this truth might make me a bad mother did not even occur to me, but I certainly never shared this conversation with anyone.

In *The New York Times*, Waldman's confession is wound around the topic of sex after children, or rather the lack of it, as she discovers in conversations with other mothers in Mommy and Me groups: "Why of all the women in the room, am I the only one who has not made the erotic transition a good mother is supposed to make? Why am I the only one incapable of placing her children at the center of her passionate universe?" I did not know what defined the good mother vs. the bad mother a year ago when I first read this essay, and I have even less of an idea now. Though the image that comes to mind when I read the words, "good mother," is Mary, of course, the Virgin Mother, holding her son adoringly on her lap, and no one should go there. But I see what Waldman is getting at. Personally I think placing your children at the center of your passionate universe is a creepy notion: children don't want that kind of pressure, there are too many responsibilities that come with being the center of another's passions. But for me, the essay takes its most interesting turn when she carries this unchanged passion for her husband to another level: "Because if I were to lose one of my children, God forbid, even if I lost all my children, God forbid, I would still have him, my husband. But my imagination simply fails me when I try to picture a future beyond my husband's death. Of course I would have to live. I have four children, a mortgage, work to do. But I can imagine no joy without my husband."

One of my favorite classes in college was a class that studied the difference between Catholicism and Buddhism. I still have the text book we used full of my notes and highlighting. I still remember the paper I wrote on the three truths of Buddha: impermanence (*anitya*), suffering (*duhkha*), and not-self (*anatman*), with a particular focus on the truth of impermanence. I had been raised in the protestant church, which like Catholicism, promises its followers an eternal life of salvation after death. It is a heavy promise that instills both peace and fear: peace in heaven for those who abide by God's laws, fear of hell for those who break them. Like Buddhists, much of life for Catholics is filled with suffering, this is undeniable, but the critical difference is that Catholics believe that God is the only force who can truly end suffering; whereas the Buddhists believe that the end of suffering can only be found within our own minds. In Catholicism you have to die first in order to see the light, in Buddhism it can only happen when one is very much alive.

Up until the age of nineteen I believed that when I died I would live in paradise with God, with my family and my friends, and with all the pets I had buried over the years in the field behind my grandmother's house. It was a beautiful and tidy picture of an afterlife free of loss and pain. But during the course of this class, I kept returning to the concept of impermanence, it whispered its terrible truth to me long after class was over, I roamed around campus contemplating mortality and its subsequent feeling of emptiness—not a frightening emptiness, my professor told us, but a calm emptiness. Think of an empty bowl, she said, a bowl sitting on a window ledge in early morning. Note your desire to want to fill the bowl. You imagine filling it with fruit, rocks, water, flowers, candles. But before you go out to the store or into your garden to gather these things, wait, let some time pass; what you may come to find is the bowl is just as beautiful empty as it is filled, perhaps even more beautiful. When I called my father, a man raised in the Episcopalian Church, and shared with him this strange discovery, he had me repeat the bowl analogy a few times, then he told me he hadn't anticipated a twenty-five thousand dollar education uprooting my entire belief system. Then he damned liberal art education and told me he loved me and not to worry because everything would straighten itself out. But when I hung up the phone it was all still waiting for me, impermanence, emptiness, that bowl.

The truth that everything changes, everything deteriorates, everything dies, I understood this before of course, but in a different guise: permanence disguised as impermanence, impermanence disguised as permanence. Yes, your grandfather is dead in that coffin, but his death isn't really permanent because there's the afterlife. So death wasn't really death at all, in fact, it was simply a separation, a break to be endured until one's own death. Here impermanence is fuzzy, open to interpretation, at once solid then suddenly shaky and loose. In Buddhism impermanence is literal. Ajahn Chah, a Thai monk, writes:

> Wanting to be different would be as foolish as wanting a duck to be a chicken. When you see that that's impossible; that a duck has to be a duck, that a chicken has to be a chicken and that bodies have to get old and die, you will find strength and energy. However much you want the body to go on and last for a long time, it won't do that.

I could not comprehend how acceptance, a daily breaking down of deep-rooted patterns of comfort and safety, could actually bring peace. The lesson now was to empty the bowl of all worldly attachments, of everything I had known and relied on and refill it, or perhaps just leave it empty.

When I looked at my future husband, a good, Catholic boy who attended Mass every Sunday in our small college town, it suddenly felt different; the way I had loved him, the depth of it, the abandon, the heart pounding passion of it had suddenly changed, it was still sweet, but there was also something somber about it now, less drastic, less extreme. I could not explain it to him or to anyone, I could hardly understand it myself. In old love letters written in high school I had contemplated a life without him, describing the same crushing joylessness Waldman describes, the same impossibility of ever loving again, of a life not really being a life, but a daily grind of meaningless rituals and misery. *I will love you forever*, I wrote in one letter, *I will not smile, I will not laugh, I will not go to Bob Pascal's keg party this weekend, I will stay home in my room, look at your picture, and stay up writing to you all night long.* I re-read these old letters with both embarrassment and awe;

I find the writer endearing, melodramatic, I hardly recognize her at first, but then I remember her, the girl who believed she would die without the boy.

It was Waldman's confession, in *The New York Times* essay, that the death of her children was more imaginable to her than the death of her husband that set off the real outrage in mothers across the country who accused her of not only being unstable, but worse, unfit to mother. The death of one's child is the number one taboo of motherhood. A taboo so terrible, so unimaginable in fact, that if dared spoken is only whispered, followed by knocking on wood, salt tossed over the shoulder, "chas veshalom," uttered by my Jewish friends, and spitting, like my Greek friends, who spit to ward off bad luck. But I found Waldman's confession normal, a bit of hyperbole perhaps, but natural, understandable, and not necessarily healthy. I do not mean the part about imagining the death of one's children, but the part about a life without her husband. It reminded me of that young girl who used to write those love letters of anguish, of physical longing, of crippling need, of the truest, deepest love ever known to mankind. This kind of love scares me now, it is a high-stakes love, an all-or-nothing love, a hormone-driven love that is unconditional only under the most perfect of conditions; in a sense it is the embodiment of two wrongs making a right.

Who can sustain such a love? Who would want to?

Perhaps Waldman's confession spoke to me directly because for so many years I felt the same way as her, and to not allow myself to feel that same devastation, that same terror at the imaginings of my life without my husband in it, has been an on-going exercise. An exercise linked with that Buddhist truth of impermanence (apologies here to my father), of the letting go of the ego, or the self, with all its tumultuous emotions and expectations of how one should live, how one should die, how one should avoid sickness and aging and pain; in essence it is the self tirelessly trying to control all in life that is simply uncontrollable. It is in the letting go that the Buddhist believes that we wake up. And like waking up from a dream, we wake up from the confusion, from the unbearable fear that might be the loss of your children or maybe it is the loss of your husband, either way, to be free of that fear and to simply be in a state of peace and acceptance and live your life unencumbered in the moment, in the right now, is the reward of this daily exercise.

But I fail often at this exercise. I watch my husband and daughter work on a puzzle. It is a *Dora the Explorer* puzzle with extra large pieces for ages 3+. My daughter has completed the puzzle many times on her own, but now she wants my husband's help. It turns out he is not very helpful; I watch as he tries to press pieces together that clearly do not fit, I think perhaps he is joking, but then I see he is not. I study my daughter's expression as she realizes that the picture forming on the floor is lopsided, and that Dora is missing the bottom half of her face; her eyes widen, then her brow furrows. She stands up, her hands grasp onto her little hips, and she reprimands him: *No, Daddy!* He looks at her with an expression of genuine surprise: *What?* She points to the jumbled mess he has made, then he laughs. She is not laughing, her face is frozen in anger, in reproof, but when he reaches for her and tickles her, her face breaks open into giggles of delight and the two of them fall on top of the puzzle.

I sit on the couch and feel it coming, like the beginnings of a fever, when deep within the flesh, within the cells of your body a signal is read that something doesn't feel right. I feel this sweet moment slowly disappear under the terrible weight of an old, nagging fear, that fear of life without my husband, of knowing if he should die tomorrow I will never love as deeply again, I will never experience a joy like this, without him my life and the life of my daughter will be defined by absences: the absence of his arms, his hands, his legs, his gorgeous face, his voice, his kindness, his perfect love; the impermanence of him, the imagining of it, is enough to make me want to throw up.

And what happens to a perfectly wonderful evening with my family, when I resist the truth of impermanence, when I hold on too tightly, clinging to my husband for dear life, inviting the fear into our house without a fight, offering it a cocktail and a comfortable place to sit? The night is ruined, and I run over to that bowl on the window ledge and puke my guts out.

But there was one time when I didn't fail.

I am in the hospital but I do not recognize the room. There are tubes running into my arms, up between my legs, I look up at two bags of what must be blood hanging like animal parts above my bed; I do not know what day it is, but I do remember this, I am a mother now. I remember my daughter's red face seconds after her birth and my husband's smile before he was rushed out of the room. Dr. Edelman leans over me, her face close to mine, I feel her cold hands press firmly on either side of my face. She keeps one hand on me and with the other she points to the strands of hair above her forehead. "You see this gray hair? I didn't have this two days ago, it's all from you, from last night. Do you know how lucky you are?" When she asks me this question it is not so much a question as a validation, a reminder that this story actually has a happy ending, though she is still unsure why.

I am held "captive" for two more weeks in the hospital, then another two in the hospital's hotel, The Helmsley, though I do not mind. Dr. Edelman is convinced I will begin to hemorrhage: "What if you're at the grocery store? Or driving on the highway?" she asks me. "Do you understand that your entire placenta was stuck in your uterus? Not a couple of small pieces, the *entire* thing." Every day she waits for the bleeding to begin, prepares me for a possible hysterectomy, and I tell her not to worry. I'm not worried, I gave birth to a healthy child, we did it, and now I have to take care of her. "Everything will be fine," I tell her, and I believe it.

Nine weeks earlier I had checked into the hospital and it did not take long before the place felt like home. I quickly learn the hospital workers by name. I know to order my lunch at breakfast time because the peanut butter and jelly sandwiches are the first to go. The nurses sit on my bed and update me on their families, their upcoming vacations, their husbands and boyfriends. My husband sleeps on a small chair that pulls out into a futon; we nickname it "the coffin." He showers for work in the bathroom connected to my room. We play Scrabble on warm August Saturday afternoons while the world outside the two windows of my room continues on without me. I begin to receive mail at the hospital: 3rd Floor Greenberg Pavilion, Room 305. I discover we are allowed to order out! We order dinners from a diner, *Angels,* that scramble eggs well-done, exactly how I like them. Every day I am wheeled down to the 2nd floor on a stretcher to listen to the baby's heart. Sometimes I wait in the hallway for 20 or 30 minutes on the stretcher before they are ready for me; it gets cold because I am wearing a hospital gown. Finally a nurse whispers in my ear, "Have your husband bring you pajamas, you don't need to wear that hideous gown all the time." My husband goes to the Gap and buys me extra large yoga pants and a white t-shirt, I feel like I a new woman.

On the day of our daughter's birth, a man known to wince at bodily fluid and blood, my husband is brave; he coaches my breathing and cuts the umbilical cord with the same ease and experience as tying a shoe. He holds our daughter, all five pounds of her, and that smile of his, it is the same smile he gave me when we were fifteen on that warm afternoon in May, standing on the hill overlooking the baseball field at Episcopal High School. I see that day in my mind perfectly: I stood next to my father who smoked a cigar, and my future husband walked right up to me and said, "hello." I watched him walk away, I couldn't believe he had the courage to talk to me in front of my father. Then the sound of the bat smacking a ball, and my father, the cigar wedged between his teeth, wrapped his arm around me as he laughed. It was my brother who hit the homerun, the last one he would ever hit, but I didn't see it, I was still watching that fifteen-year-old boy walk away.

For the next three hours while my doctor works on me, I stare up at the ceiling and ignore the straps pinning my arms down to the bed, the tug of hands on my hips, hands extracting pieces of placenta from my uterus; I ignore the crew of doctors that stream in and circle around me like ghosts; I ignore the voices, the tension, the sound of soft shoes sliding back and forth quickly across the floor. I do not see light, I do not pray to God, I see my husband's smile, I imagine his hands pressed against me, but there is so much pain now, seeping through the loosening haze of the epidural, I almost laugh that pain could be like this, really like *this.* I glance up at my doctor, I can see it in her face, she thinks I am dying and she's not sure she can stop it. I look for my husband but he's not here, then I feel a surge in my chest, a scream of injustice, of fear, it rushes up my throat, it is the scream of every mother who has bled to death after childbirth, it is horrible, the sound of it, the shaking rage of it, of knowing you will not watch your child grow up, that life will go on without you. But before it reaches my mouth I bite my lips together, I stare up at the ceiling light, at the shadows dancing, and I breathe. I quiet the scream, I will it away, I will it away; it won't help me, it will only break me. There is a sudden clarity in this instant when I finally understand what it is that I have to contend with; thoughts of my husband, my daughter, they are gone, forgotten, it is the only way; this moment is the only thing that makes sense to me now, it is all my mind has room for. I am alone, I accept this and there is peace to be found here. Acceptance is not surrender, in fact it is work; I am tired but no longer scared. There is still so much work to do.

Big Girl Pants

I lie on my mat in yoga class and think of nothing. My eyes are closed but I feel the presence of a body preparing to sit next to me on my right; and a few minutes later I feel the presence of another body to my left. When I hear the instructor's voice I sit up. I look to my right, sitting cross-legged, quite close to me, is a woman who must be eight months pregnant, her hands rest on her large belly. Then I look to my left to find another woman, also sitting quite close to me, large with pregnancy, her hands rest on her knees. It is not a pre-natal class, nor is it a crowded class, the rest of the people, both men and women (who are not pregnant, at least not visibly), are spread out comfortably in the room; suddenly I am not comfortable. It would be awkward and perhaps unkind to pick up my mat and move away from them, so I remain where I am, sandwiched in between two of the most pregnant women in New York City.

The instructor introduces herself, April is her name (naturally), and she walks over and squats close to the floor in front of me, though it is the two pregnant women whom she addresses. She asks them how far along they are (one is 36 weeks, the other 34) and for the next few minutes they chat about certain poses they should not do: head stand, lotus and any other pose which requires pressure on the stomach, lower back, or head. Then April looks at me, perhaps thinking I feel left out. "Clearly, you are not pregnant!" I smile and shake my head no, hoping she will go away now, but she has not moved. "I mean, you don't look pregnant, but you could be," she pats me on the knee. "No," I assure her. "I'm not."

It is December, parkas and fur and heavy scarves and ponchos disguise all of us, but inside this studio we wear very little, and I cannot help but stare at these two women as they move gracefully through the vinyasas. I am surprised by how well they manage the postures; despite their size, there is very little that they cannot do. Their long, white arms cradle their bellies as their backs arch and legs bend; I imagine the babies inside their bellies mirroring their mothers' positions, their tiny backs stretched, legs bent, heads bowed low.

As I stand up tall, stretching my arms up over my head, the pregnant woman to my right brushes my arm with her hand; *Sorry*, she whispers. *It's okay*, I whisper back. As I sweep my arms down to the ground I feel tears slide down my face, falling onto the mat, I rub them away with my toes.

My daughter calls to me in the middle of the night. I go to her. I sit on the floor next to her bed and run my finger across her cheek. Her eyes stare up at the ceiling.

I have a baby, she whispers, smoothing her hands over her tummy.

How is the baby? I ask. She presses her fingers over her mouth.

Shhh. Don't talk, the baby is sleeping.

The real baby is 22 weeks old now. It has grown to about 12 inches long and weighs one pound. Its tongue is fully formed and if it is a girl her internal reproductive organs have developed. The mother will notice more movement now, quick jerking motions indicate the baby has the hiccups. The baby responds to touch and sounds; its heart rate increases at the sound of its mother's voice.

***

It is Christmas. I meet a friend for coffee and she asks me the second question I have come to fear most.

"When are you telling people?" She begins.

"Telling people what?"

"Don't be coy. You know what I'm talking about."

I think on it for a minute.

"I'm not going to tell people," I say.

"You are just going to show up with a baby, out of the blue?"

"Yes!" I think of those mad storks on the walls at the

hospital in Indiana.

She studies me for a few minutes. She is a dear friend. She lost a baby a few years ago, right after his birth; he was her first child.

"Eventually you're going to have to put your big-girl pants on, you know that," she says.

"God, I hate those pants."

"I know."

I have been wondering why we have children. I find that it is not a question that invites an easy response. As with all experiments in my life I begin with my husband while he is trying to read the paper. He is like our daughter in his ability to transcend time, space, and the sound of his name when he is busy; and I am like our daughter in my impulsiveness and in my worship of the Right Now. He peers up at me and asks me to repeat the question; I repeat it and he says, "You know..." then pauses, allowing me to fill in the spaces. When I do not fill in the spaces he adds, "It's fun." Fun? Obviously this is not a sufficient answer so I ask again and he tells me he will get back to me later after he thinks on it. I do not pry because I know how he feels, I don't have a profound answer either.

Perhaps our increasing life span or the fact that more and more women wait until their 30's, 40's and 50's to have babies, maybe all of this extra time leaves us in places of reflection that biology never meant for us to visit: perhaps we were never meant to ask that question. I imagine people five thousand years ago did not ask the question because the answer was obvious: to maintain the human race (Shakespeare's, *The Tempest*, comes to mind with its beast Caliban who would like to copulate with Miranda in order to "people the island with Calibans" for no other reason than lust and spreading his seed). When I ask my mother why she and her peers in the 60's had babies so young, she says: "Because we had sex without protection."

My maternal grandmother is 80, a mother of three, a grandmother of seven, a great-grandmother of one (and soon two), a North Carolinian, and a devoted wife to my grandfather of 56 years. I ask her why she had children. She pauses for a second or two. "Well, that's just what you did." She laughs, she is sweet but not naïve, she knows I'm looking for a juicier answer, but she doesn't have one. "And I'm sure glad I did," she adds.

From a young age I knew that I wanted to be a mother. I was a child who loved babies, I loved holding them, I loved how they smelled, I loved the whole idea of dressing them up in bonnets and tiny shoes and carrying them around on my hip. I believe this desire was both an embodiment of instinct and legacy. My mother and my grandmothers were proud mothers, kind and strong, and at least from my perspective balanced their superhero roles with the realities of life effortlessly. Of course it helped that the world of the 70's in which I grew up was not a kid-centric environment like the one we have created for our children today. My brother and I left home on our bikes in the mornings and returned home before sundown, sometimes we stopped back home for a quick lunch, oftentimes we did not. Who wouldn't co-exist amicably with an 8-hour break from each other every day? Homecomings in the evenings were welcomed, delicious food was prepared and waiting, and bedtime stories were read with enthusiasm and vigor. In essence, my brother and I conformed to our parents' lifestyle, not the other way around. Like I said, it was the 70's, my mother was reading Michener, not *The Happiest Toddler on the Block*. We were brought along to late-night dinners and cocktail parties; we fell asleep in restaurant booths, on laps, on couches, in the backseats of cars. Our parents stayed out late and slept late, and we learned to cook breakfast for ourselves, and at some point realized a twenty dollar bill from my father's bedside table would buy a very nice breakfast at the diner down the street. Summers were spent at the beach in Ocean City, Maryland. We lived on my father's 48' Egg Harbor sport fisherman boat. Days were unstructured, often unsupervised, pleas of boredom and injustice were largely ignored, which had the brilliant effect of shutting us up. Activities included fishing, swimming, fishing, cutting bait, watching other people fish, crabbing, and more fishing. I grew up in a grown-up world of smoking, drinking, sunbathing without sunblock, endless games of Scrabble and bridge, a lot of Ritz crackers and port cheese, and adult conversation: divorce, sex, adultery, and money. I don't remember anything ever said about motherhood or children.

During the other seasons of the year, I have fond memories of ice skating on the pond in front of my grandmother's house with my mother and father, playing baseball with my father and brother in the backyard, weekend trips to Colonial Williamsburg where we made candles and skillet bread, Halloween parties (my mother hand-sewed all of my costumes), and family games of Yahtzee and Monopoly. My parents somehow achieved a balance between their identities as parents and their identities as adults with interests beyond us, guilt-free.

The notion of childlessness was something more shocking to me than to my parents or to their friends, perhaps because I was a child and could not imagine a woman and man *out there* not wanting one of *me*. Even today I can remember every one of my parents' friends (and their names) who had no children, I can remember my incessant questioning of my mother as to why, and I can remember her nonchalant attitude about the entire concept.

My husband and I were married six years before we had our daughter. My desire to have a baby hit me on the morning of my thirtieth birthday, it hit me hard — like that moment of panic and bewilderment when you realize you have lost your wallet. How could this have happened? We were living in a one-bedroom apartment in New York City at the time, and I sat up in bed and wanted a baby. This was not a want for the future, it was a want for right now, for that very instant; I wanted a baby to hold in my arms, to wrap up in a blanket and to love, to love lavishly. The day before, when I was still twenty-nine, I had no inkling of this, no warning, no signs of how my life would be changed in less than twenty-four hours. It felt deeply unfair and cruel, and yet there was an undeniable element of excitement in this sudden desire, it felt very much like my first love for Sean Cassidy that wasn't rational, and there were times that staring up at the four-foot poster of him on my bedroom wall evoked in me such passion that I would press my mouth against his for minutes at a time until my nose hurt from the pressure of the wall. Then there were other times when it felt odd, confusing, so different from the day that I carefully hung the poster: where was this going? Did we really have a future together? And that bulge in his pants, below his belt buckle, that hit me right at eye level, did I *really* want to know what that was all about? When these questions became too much, when I felt that I was in over my head, I would leave my room and retreat to the safety of my mother's lap where her skin was always tan and soft, and life was uncomplicated.

The initial reason why I wanted a baby, I have no idea really. Perhaps the memories of sitting on my mother's lap as she painted her toenails or read the paper evoked in me the desire to try and repeat history, or maybe it had something to do with hormones, like those same pre-adolescent sex hormones that kicked in on the day I fell in love with Sean Cassidy. But unlike my goal to marry Sean, my desire for a baby matured out of its reckless first beginnings and transformed into something strong, focused, so determined that at times it made my entire body ache. It would take two more years, fertility treatments, and three miscarriages before I looked down at our daughter's glorious body asleep in my arms.

I call my mother and ask her about a childless couple she and my father used to boat with in the 70's. After her initial shock that I actually remember the name of the couple, she tells me they were divorced years ago and they both live in Florida somewhere.

"Did they divorce because they didn't have children?" I ask.

My mother laughs. "Lord, no. He drank too much and she found Jesus."

There is a website dedicated to people without children, it is called Childfree.net.

Who are we? The question headlines its title page. I am told that Childfree.net consists of a group of adults who have chosen not to have children:

> We choose to call ourselves 'childfree' rather than 'childless' because we feel the term 'childless' implies that we're missing something we want—and we aren't. We consider ourselves childfree—free of the loss of personal freedom, money, time, and energy that having children

requires.

What draws me to read further is not to learn more about these obvious losses, but to understand the purpose of their website: "The disapproving stares and cries of 'How can you not want children?!' often send us into a form of hiding. We feel like freaks and don't realize exactly how many of us there are and exactly how much information is actually out there. This site attempts to remedy that problem."

Freaks in hiding, now this is interesting to me; and the notion that the number of "freaks" out there is unknown, is yet to be discovered, gives this whole concept a mysterious air, *The Planet of the Apes* pops into my mind. And what kind of information, exactly, are they gathering? They list different websites, such as overpopulation.org, that pose the question: "Is it ethical to have children?" There is nokidding.net, a self-described social club full of childless people, begun in Canada in 1984. The club features anywhere from three to eight smoke-free social activities a month that range from hiking and barbecues to wine and cheese parties. This website features a list of its members' testimonials. *Laurie* remembers being a child of eight and knowing she would never have children:

> I spotted my mother struggling with heavy boxes of fruit as she tried to place them in the back of a truck. 'Why does Mom work so hard all the time?' The thought echoed incessantly through my mind. It did not seem fair to see my mother constantly working so hard for long hours. My mother's sacrifice of herself for her family gave me no desire to follow in her footsteps...I sat down on the piano bench and began to practice my lesson. 'Stop that awful noise!' My father's voice boomed from the easy chair in the living room.

There is *Gouri's* story, a woman comfortable with her decision not to have children, to exist within that "important contingent of adults: aunts and uncles and godparents," and to tolerate the constant "inquisitions" such a choice invites.

If you live in India you get used to total strangers on trains asking you even before they know your name: 'Any issue?' Which is an archaic expression for: 'Got any kids?' And when you answer, 'No,' they almost always cluck in sympathy. If you're a woman, and another woman asks you the question, then she will go on to ask: 'Married how many years? Been to a doctor?' As a person who has chosen not to have children, you then have two options: Either you chicken out and mumble, 'Yes, I've been to a doctor, but I can't have kids.' So that the sympathetic clucking goes on for a while, and then she leaves you alone. Or, you take the tougher option — if you're up to being lectured, harangued, questioned, and finally labeled — and say pleasantly: 'I've decided not to have children.'

There are other reasons given in other testimonials, such as the dangers of passing on genetic diseases, the threat of nuclear extinction, the inherent cruelty of children, and a general dislike of miniature adults who shit themselves. But as I read through the other testimonials from this and other websites the same themes reoccur: money and the environment. Children are expensive (it will cost an estimated $843,508 to raise a child to 18 years of age), and they damage the environment by adding to pollution.

Back at Childfree.net there is a "potpourri page" with suggested books to read such as, *The Childless Revolution; Families of Two; and Cheerfully Childless: The Humor Book for Those Who Hesitate to Procreate.* There is a list of celebrity/notable childfrees: Stockard Channing, George Clooney, Linda Evans, Oprah, Dolly Parton, Dr. Seuss, and Georgia O'Keefe, among others. It is only because I am now a "freak" in my own right that I understand why Dolly Parton's childlessness is relevant: Dolly Parton is a far cry from *The Planet of the Apes*, and because our culture worships celebrities and their clothes, their homes and their lifestyles, her choice makes childlessness chic.

Our first phone conversation with Norah took place last April. I had been given suggested topics of conversation by the psychologist at the surrogacy agency in order to make the phone meeting less awkward, but we didn't need it. The moment I heard Norah's voice I knew she was the one to help us have a baby, and what was even more of a surprise is how much I liked her. I liked her voice, I liked her easygoing nature, I liked her laugh; so much of human connection is visceral. Toward the end of the conversation, when we had covered the practical points and the logistics of our partnership, I found myself presenting a subject that neither Norah nor the psychologist had mentioned: and that was the question of why we wanted another child when we already had a healthy child. I stumbled over my words, I was ineloquent, I repeated myself and spoke in circles like someone tortured by guilt, until Norah finally interrupted me.

"You don't need to explain why you want a baby, Ashley," she said. "I understand."

***

I take the trash out, it is late, after ten o'clock. As I close the door to the trash room I see that my neighbor is walking down the hall toward me. I feel my pulse speed up, I quickly scan my escape options, but there are none. She, on the other hand, is glad that she has run into me because something has been on her mind.

"Is there any possible way that you will be able to breast feed?" she asks.

I do not know how to answer her; she must read this in my expression.

"The only reason why I ask is that when I was pregnant with my children my mother actually gained the exact same amount of weight as I did and ..." Her voice trails off as I begin to back away toward my apartment door. "Or perhaps you could hire someone to breastfeed the baby," she adds.

"Like a wet nurse?" I ask. Good God.

"Well, yes," she says. "I've done a little research and there are actual milk banks for situations — for people, like you."

For people like me? I inch closer to my apartment.

"How is the — the woman?" she asks, referring to Norah.

"She's great. She's fine, everybody's fine."

She shakes her head. "I just can't imagine giving up a baby," she says, staring at me, squinting her eyes as if looking for the answer within me.

"But it's not her baby." The words just come out, forcibly, like gasping for breath, and I want to kick myself. What I had meant to say was: "Yes, amazing, isn't it?" or something along those lines, vague and noncommittal.

"This is obviously a sensitive topic for you," she says. She suddenly seems irritated with me, as if I have affronted her. She crosses her arms, waiting for a reply.

"No, no, it's fine. Thank you — I'll check into the milk bank. Well, good-night," I say. And quickly escape into my apartment, locking the door behind me.

Almost Home

It is the end of February and the baby is 29 weeks old now, he weighs about three pounds and is measuring around 11 inches long. At this stage the mother often feels fluttering and twitching because the baby gets the hiccups frequently as he begins to drink amniotic fluid, preparing his lungs for birth when he must breathe air.

We receive a letter from the surrogacy agency's Guidance Team entitled: *Almost Home! Weeks 27-40*. It is a three-page letter, typed onto lavender paper, full of tips and a long check-list to guide us through these final weeks before the birth and into the final stages at the hospital. Since September we have received notes from "The Guidance Team," notes containing tips and advice on interacting with one's surrogate mother, notes I have, for the most part, skimmed over and thrown away. This letter I read more carefully.

It begins:

> These next 13 weeks can be stressful for all parties. Your surrogate mother will likely have much less energy and mobility. Her focus shifts to "having your baby" and getting her life back. You may hear less excitement in her voice and more frustration. This is normal and it does not mean that she regrets helping you. She is just beginning to feel "finished." Together our job is to support her desire to be "done" but encourage her to rest and have a full-term pregnancy. We are all on "her" team. Let your counselor know your concerns.

What follows is a list of 19 tips and "considerations" to go over before admittance to the hospital. Many cover the practicalities of the situation such as: discussing the "birth experience" with your surrogate mother, establishing a contact plan so that your surrogate mother can reach you at any time of day or night in case labor begins unexpectedly, understanding hospital policies about ID bands, "rooming-in" policies and what to do if a C-section should occur, acquiring a birth certificate with the hospital clerk and delivering it to County Birth Records, obtaining a certified birth certificate in order to get a passport, getting a handwritten note from the doctor in order to give to the airline in case documentation is needed for the newborn, and purchasing an approved car seat.

Somewhere in the middle of the list the practicalities shift to points of etiquette:

- **Under NO circumstances should you leave town before your surrogate mother is discharged from the hospital** (local couples may want to discuss exceptions).

- The Center for Surrogacy Parenting staff can send flowers from you to your surrogate mother if you request it. If not requested, CSP will assume that you are taking care of the flowers directly.

- **It is IMPORTANT that your surrogate mother gets some alone time with the baby/babies if she desires.** She may not feel comfortable asking. This does not provoke bonding, but rather allows her to conclude her relationship with the baby. This helps her finish her job and turn the parenting over to you. It is nice if you offer her this chance. Handing her the baby demonstrates your trust and sensitivity.

- After the birth you will follow the baby to watch the bath, and first exams. Please check back with your surrogate mother often to give her a report and see how she is doing. Some surrogate mothers feel left out and lost at this point and remain concerned about you and the baby.

• Take lots of pictures — pictures help surrogate mother re-experience what happened so fast and allows them to better complete the emotional process. Plus, pictures are fun to share and help others celebrate. A lack of pictures is a regret.

• Post birth contact — it is difficult when contact changes from very frequent (prior to birth) to infrequent or no contact after leaving the hospital. Our best advice is to call when you arrive home with the baby and tell your surrogate mother when you will call next. If comfortable, invite her to call if she wants — she knows you will be adjusting to a new schedule. Let communication gradually decrease as she recovers and gets back to her routine. Abrupt changes in communication can create misunderstandings.

Perhaps it is the tone of this letter I dislike, or the hint of condescension in reminding me to be courteous and thoughtful and humane, or maybe it is the portrayal of the surrogate mother as fragile and needy that puts me off, someone with whom we must tread lightly. I do not know this surrogate mother, I do not recognize her; there is nothing about her character that even resembles Norah.

What this letter seems to reflect is the same problem I am finding in the world beyond my safe friends: they're getting it all wrong.

Of course I have done nothing to correct the misconceptions, to set the record straight, to campaign for a clearer understanding of who Norah is and the scope of what she is doing for me and for my husband and daughter. I have not done this because at this point I do not know how.

No, that is not true. I do know how. But it demands a level of honesty and strength that I do not possess.

At least not today.

I find myself stuck between my stubborn nature and my knowledge of what it means to do the right thing. I cling to privacy, it is a large part of who I am, but in order to be understood, in order to do the right thing and to stop hiding Norah, I must let that go, privacy must be relinquished. But how do I do that? It seems that once you open up, once you reveal what is private and personal with one and all, the line between what is private and what is open territory is gone, what was once sacred suddenly becomes shared, consumed, and ultimately changed. There is risk in sharing beliefs, dreams, life's disappointments. I have always felt this risk acutely. It is not that I have been burned or betrayed any more than the average person; perhaps it has less to do with trust and more to do with perspective, a natural tendency to position myself as observer to confessions, to the outpouring of emotion, and how often I have watched and actually felt something lost during the discloser. When you watch those infamous Barbara Walters interviews with celebrities and politicians, do you not feel that at some point during the questioning, during the inevitable admittance of heartbreak and disappointment, amidst the tears, that the original feelings of pain have somehow been cheapened, compromised, hollowed out? What was once raw and true is now as common place as the Tide commercial that follows during the commercial break. Is it possible to share one's story, to share one's dramas in the light of its original unveiling, without losing something?

I place the letter from the Guidance Team in the drawer. I sit at my desk and feel the crunch of time closing in on me. If the pregnancy continues to go smoothly, which I know it will, the baby will arrive in a little less than two months. I feel a panic as I realize that I have not told my daughter's teacher about the baby, nor have I told the director of her school. Her pre-school is a close-knit school, a Montessori school, one which emphasizes community and family and sharing. I wonder if my daughter has mentioned to her teacher news about the real baby or about the baby growing in her tummy, or perhaps both. I pick up the phone to call her teacher and make an appointment.

Angry Lion

In Andre Dubus's short story, *The Winter Father*, Peter describes the day his six-year-old daughter suffers her first injury.

> In early spring a year ago: he still had not taken the storm windows off the screen doors; he was bringing his lunch to the patio, he did not know that Kathi was following him, and holding his plate and mug he had pushed the door open with his shoulder, stepped outside, heard the crash and her scream, and turned to see her gripping then pulling the long shard from her cheek. She got it out before he reached her. He picked her up and pressed his handkerchief to the wound, midway between her eye and throat, and held her as he phoned the doctor who said he would meet them at the hospital and do the stitching himself because it was cosmetic and that beautiful face should not be touched by residents...
>
> Kathi lay on the car seat beside him and he held his handkerchief on her cheek, and in the hospital he held her hands while she lay on the table. The doctor said it would only take about four stitches and it would be better without anesthetic, because sometimes that puffed the skin and he wanted to fit the cut together perfectly, for the scar; he told this very gently to Kathi, and he said as she grew, the scar would move down her face and finally be under her jaw. Then she and Peter squeezed each other's hands as the doctor

stitched and she gritted her teeth and stared at
pain.

As I lie in bed after a long afternoon and evening in
the Lenox Hill Hospital Emergency Room with my daughter,
I think of this story. I look at the clock, it is a little after two in
the morning and I get out of bed to search for the book. Most of
my books are still in boxes from our move last year, boxes that
are stacked up high in the storage closet. Four heavy boxes full
of books I drop to the floor, dumping their contents, searching
for the book, mumbling to myself, *come on, baby*. A part of me
recognizes that I am still on an adrenaline rush, the other part of
me cares nothing about explanations or reasoning, I am desperate
to find the book, that particular story, and I sort through the boxes
and create a large mess. When I find the book, with the black and
white picture of Dubus on the cover, I study his gray beard and
kind eyes, his head leaning against his hand, and I lie down on the
floor, pressing the book against my chest, then kiss it.

"The Jackman's marriage had been adulterous and
violent," the story begins, "but in its last days, they became
a couple again, as they might have if one of them were slowly
dying." When Peter and his wife sit at the kitchen table and tell
eight-year-old David about the divorce he cries violently, begs
them not to, then escapes to his room; but Kathi does nothing. She
sits and stares at them, Peter remembers, her expression the same
as the year before when the doctor had sewn the wound on her
face closed.

I don't actually see my daughter's head slam into the
edge of the wooden locker. What I hear are her screams, and
by the time I reach her she is on her knees, her hands pressed
against her forehead, covered in blood. I hold her in my arms and
gently pull her hands away to see how bad it is: the wound is
deep, shaped like an upside-down triangle, and as blood pours
from it, it begins to look eerily like a mouth, and as the bleeding
continues the cut widens; I watch the skin spread into something
now resembling the shape of a smile. I stare at this terrible smile,
then at my daughter's mouth, frozen in a cry, unable to find the
words to tell me how much it hurts.

In the ambulance I lie on the stretcher with my daughter on top of me. Elvira, the paramedic helping us, tells me this will help calm her. She shines a flashlight in my daughter's eyes, asks her questions: *What is your name? How old are you? Does your tummy hurt?* My daughter does not answer, she only wails and stares at the blood on her hands and tilts her head back against my chest, shaking it no. Elvira asks me questions about the fall: *Did you pick her up immediately? Did she lose consciousness? Is she allergic to any medication?* Then she tries once more with my daughter: *What is your mommy's name?* Suddenly my daughter's crying calms and she tells her my name. Elvira looks at me to make sure this is right. I nod my head. Then my daughter turns to Elvira for the first time and asks her why she's wearing earrings.

In *Winter Father* Peter tries to make his children's lives normal again, he tries to veil the pain divorce has caused them:

> When they were too loud in the car or when they fought, he held onto his anger, his heart buffeted with it, and spoke calmly, as though to another man's children, for he was afraid that if he scolded as he had before, the day would be spoiled, they would not have the evening at home, that sleeping in the same house, to heal them; and they might not want to go with him the next day or two nights from now or two days.

As we sit in a holding room in the hospital, waiting for the plastic surgeon to arrive, my daughter no longer wants or needs the security of my lap. The bleeding has stopped, the horror of the fall is all but forgotten in her mind, and she pushes my arms away and walks to a chair across the room where she climbs into it and sits down with a thump, her arms stretched out on the arm rests, her legs shoot straight out over the seat. She stares at me with the coolness and pride of a child Emperor. Within seconds I am on my knees, sitting at her feet, stroking her arms as she announces, in her stream-of-consciousness manner, all the things she would like to have: bubble gum, pacifiers, earrings, a necklace, play-dates with Paul, Manon, Cayla, extra-large white marshmallows on a stick, and balloons, eight balloons, to be exact, pink ones. *Of course, of course! Anything you want, my darling,* I tell her, *anything in the world you want.* As she considers this offer I stare at the wound, I cannot help myself. There is her gorgeous face, perfect, poreless and fine, and there above her left eyebrow a grotesque hole, an opening, revealing the raw red and pink layers of fat protecting the skull, still smiling at me, more a smirk now, a reminder to me of how fragile the face is, how fragile the life.

She feels me staring at the wound and raises her hand to touch it—No! I grab her hand but she pulls it away from me and crosses her arms, turning her head away. I have hurt her pride, I have reminded her of why we are here. *What about ten balloons?* I ask. She does not answer, instead she reaches her hand down to me, signaling that I may hold it again. We sit in silence, she in the chair, me still at her feet. Then she asks me to tell her again about that clown, Looney Louie, who pulled a pair of underpants out of his hat. I tell her. *Again,* she says, *tell me again.*

At the end of *Winter Father*, Peter realizes that he and his children are happiest during the summer when they spend days at the beach:

> For on that day, a long Saturday at the beach, when he had all day felt peace and father-love and sun and salt water, he had understood why now in summer he and his children were as he had yearned for them to be in winter: they were no longer confined to car or buildings to remind them why they were there. The long beach and sea were their lawn; the blanket their home; the ice chest and thermos their kitchen.

At the end of that day as the three of them lie on the blanket Peter says, "Divorced kids go to the beach more than married ones." David replies, "I love the beach." But Kathi says nothing. "You don't like it, huh?" Peter asks her.

She took her arm away from her eyes and looked
at him. His urge was to turn away. She looked at
him for a long time; her eyes were too tender, too
wise, and he wished she could have learned both
later, and differently; in her eyes he saw the car in
winter, heard its doors closing and closing, their
talk and the sounds of the heater and engine and
tires on the road, and the places the car took them.
Then she held his hand, and closed her eyes. 'I
wish it was summer all year round,' she said. He
watched her face, rosy tan now, lightly freckled;
her small scar was already lower. Holding her
hand, he reached for David's, and closed his eyes
against the sun.

Kathi's wish for summer to never end answers her father's
declaration that divorced kids go to the beach more than married
ones, then it subtly lifts the veil of its lie. She is old enough now
to understand the power of forgetting, of changing the scenery
in an attempt to change the truth — it feels good, as good as lying
on the beach and feeling the sun dry wet skin. She would like to
lie on that blanket beneath the sun with her father and brother
forever, but experience has taught her better than to believe this
could be possible; and maybe that is the worst part of pain, the
way it unhinges one's hopes, one's beliefs in impossibilities, the
way it distorts a moment in time with a single blow. Kathi knows
that soon they must pack up the blanket, wash the sand from their
bodies, and get back into her father's car; that he must drive them
home and drop them off in front of the house he no longer shares
with them; and that summer will end and fall will begin and they
will find themselves back inside the car, watching rain fall, then
snow, listening to the heater hum, and the engine's roar.

Peter believes it is his fault that his daughter understands
this truth so soon, and it probably is. But what is to be done to
prevent it? How do we prevent marriages from ending, or the
seasons from changing, or wooden lockers from colliding with a
child's head?

What is your favorite animal? The doctor carefully slides

the needle beneath my daughter's skin. He works quickly, though meticulously, he is calm, his voice is gentle. I lie on the hospital bed along side my daughter, holding her hands as the nurse holds her head still. I watch her blue eyes dart here and there, contemplating the question. Then:

An angry lion, she snarls.

The doctor's hand continues to move across her head with the needle.

An 'angry lion'? He says. *Why?*

I feel my daughter's hands slide away from mine as she holds them up to him, shaped now like a lion's paws. *Because they roar!* She roars, an open mouth roar.

You scared me, the doctor says.

She slides her hands back beneath mine, and smiles.

Jackson

Medical science has risen to the occasion and created new avenues to parenthood alongside the more traditional family building practices. These new practices are confusing and certainly call into question how best to describe them to children. However, describe we must, so as not to break trust with our children around issues of truth. Our children deserve to know the truth about their life beginnings; they should learn it from their parents, and they should see their beginnings as natural. This book [*Mommy, Did I Grow in Your Tummy?*] is badly needed to help parents discuss the topics of birth origins with sensitivity and honesty.

> Book Review of *Mommy, Did I grow in Your Tummy?* Sharon Kaplan, B.S.W., M.S.

I am finally desperate enough to buy that children's book the surrogacy agency recommended about the childless couple Sandy and Bob, their cat Pancake, and their dog Spot. In the first packet of information from the agency that we received three years ago, an advertisement in eye-catching hot-pink for *Mommy, Did I Grow in Your Tummy?* was included. The book was published in 1992, and aside from its actual printing press in Santa Monica, California, I could only find the book through a used book dealer on the internet. Neither Barnes and Noble, Borders, or Amazon carried it.

A thin white package arrives in the mail from a bookstore

in Florida; I immediately know what it is. I quickly slide it into my purse and wait until evening when my daughter is asleep before opening it.

It is a paperback book, 28 pages long. The title, in its entirety, is: *Mommy, Did I Grow in Your Tummy? Where Some Babies Come From.* And beneath the title are the names of its author and illustrator, as well as their means of becoming mothers: Elaine R. Gordon, Ph.D., Mom Via Adoption and Kathy Clo, Mom Via Invitro.

The first page is a picture of a woman and her daughter standing in the middle of their living room looking at each other. The daughter's mouth is open, her expression one of youthful innocence: "Mommy, did I grow in your tummy?" she asks.

On the next page the scene has moved to the couch. The daughter sits in between her mother and father. This is the father's first appearance and, oddly, he seems disinterested in this most important conversation: he is reading the newspaper. But the mother is engaged, staring down lovingly at her daughter, as she begins her story.

"That's a very important question," the mother says. "I'm so glad you asked. Come sit down next to me and I'll read you a story..."

The mother tells a story of Sandy and Bob. Sandy and Bob dream of having a baby. Bob dreams of playing catch with the baby, Sandy dreams of rocking the baby to sleep. Sandy and Bob have a cat named Pancake and a dog named Spot. Though Sandy and Bob love each other very much and have a wonderful life, something is missing. The Bakers down the street just had a baby and Sandy's cousins, Ann and Sam, just had a baby; even Sugar, the neighborhood dog just had a litter of puppies. Sandy and Bob decide to make a baby.

But no matter how hard they try, no baby comes.

So Sandy and Bob go to a doctor, a Dr. Preston, who tells them that there are many ways to make a baby. The illustrations show men and women, sperms and eggs, and growing fetuses inside wombs, as traditional and invitro fertilization are explained. "Doctors can be pretty helpful but sometimes a mom and dad need even more help," the mother explains. And things get a bit complicated as the method of egg and **sperm donor** are explained.

> A mom might not have an egg to join with the dad's sperm. But she can still grow a baby in her body. When this happens, another woman, called an egg donor, can help by donating or giving her egg to meet and join with the dad's sperm.

Next to the pictures of a mother and father is a picture of a woman in a knee-length skirt and sensible shoes holding a book entitled, "Egg Donor." On the next page the same scenario is explained, but this time with the sperm donor (a man in nice brown trousers and a tie). Next comes the surrogacy option; I pay close attention to this explanation:

> Some moms can't make or grow a baby. It just doesn't work no matter how hard she tries. When this happens a mom and dad can get help from a **surrogate**. Surrogate is a hard word but it's easy to understand... What usually happens is the mom and dad choose a very special woman to be the surrogate. The doctor puts the dad's sperm into the surrogate so she can grow the baby inside her for the mom and dad.

What she describes is traditional surrogacy, not gestational surrogacy; it does not apply to me. Adoption is the final method in the mother's story, it is explained with the least amount of biology.

But I am still wondering about Sandy and Bob.

Then, "Guess what!" the mother says at the bottom of page 25. And on page 26 the good news is finally revealed: Sandy and Bob have a baby. The illustration is of Sandy and Bob and their new baby girl, with Pancake and Spot standing up on their hind legs smiling at the new addition to their family.

"I'm not sure which way they decided to grow their family," the mother says. "But it really doesn't matter because they ended up with their dream — a wonderful, wonderful baby."

I turn the page, it is the last page of the book, and we are back on the couch. The mother and the little girl embrace and the father looks at them, smiling, his newspaper neatly folded next to him.

I re-read the book.

I read it again.

I think about that day at the surrogacy agency's office two years ago when the psychological counselor asked: "What do you intend to tell your child about his or her unique beginnings?"

I remember our blank expressions.

I read the book one more time.

I realize that I did not buy this book to read to my unborn child years from now, I bought it for myself, for today, in the hopes that a book written for children with simple vocabulary and nice pictures would explain to me how to explain this "unique beginning" to myself. Instead, I find myself exactly in the same place I was before: stuck in a world of abstractions and uncertainty.

I turn back to page 27 of the children's book and read it again: "I'm not sure which way they decided to grow their family, but it really doesn't matter because they ended up with their dream — a wonderful, wonderful baby."

If it doesn't really matter, then why write the book? And years from now, when our unborn child is old enough to understand where babies come from, what if the question never comes up? Do I bring it up? According to Sharon Kaplan, the child expert, "our children deserve to know the truth about their life beginnings." I try to put myself in our unborn child's shoes. I think of my mother and father, of my life with them, of everything they gave me, and the truth is I wouldn't really care how they got me here; the facts wouldn't change anything. At least I don't think the facts would change anything. Maybe this is not a fair assessment, for I came into the world the "normal" way; perhaps if I had been adopted or born with the help of a surrogate, like my unborn child, I would feel differently.

I am more confused than before. Not to mention the fact that I will never know how Sandy and Bob got their baby.

But then again, maybe it wasn't any of my business. And maybe that's the point.

***

The phone rings. I listen to it ring and check the caller ID: Unknown Caller. I have no choice but to answer calls from Unknown Callers these days in case it might be Norah or the hospital in Indianapolis. It is not Norah or the hospital in Indianapolis, it is a cousin of mine. We are not close. I don't think we have spoken on the phone, ever, and I am wondering who gave her my phone number. She is calling because she is concerned over what she is going to tell her children about my situation.

"My situation?" I ask.

"The woman — the woman who's having your baby. I've been going over it in my head and I have no idea how to explain it to my kids," she says. "I've really hit a wall here."

In Buddhism there is a practice referred to as "giving and taking." In this practice one aspires to attain enlightenment in order to help another; it trains the mind to feel only compassion when confronted with a jackass. In order to attain such compassion one must go through several phases: 1) one must meditate, calming the body, contemplating enlightenment, 2) one then visualizes one's own mother with the understanding that over the course of many re-births everyone has been each other's mother at one point, enabling one to extend the compassion one feels towards one's mother to other people, and 3) finally, when one feels the compassion and then resolves to extend it, the practice of taking and giving begins. "Taking happens with the in-breath. Giving happens with the out-breath." Gyalwa Gendun Gyatso, the second Dalai Lama, writes:

> Consider how all friends and relatives, having been your mother again and again in previous lives, have shown you the same kindness as has your present mother. In each previous life, they, as your mother (of that life) have shown

you all the kindness of a mother, and in that respect are every bit as deserving of your love and appreciation as is the mother of this life. Contemplate over and over how they were kind mothers, until the mere sight of any of them fills your heart with joy and appreciation. Then consider how, enmeshed in suffering, they are barren of true happiness. Continue meditating in this way until compassion unable to bear their pitiable state arises...meditate like this until love and compassion arise, and then meditate upon 'giving and taking' — taking the immediate and indirect cause of their anger, distortion and unhappiness and giving them the cause of peace and joy.

The inevitable question that arises from this practice is what to do if your present mother is a witch from hell, but luckily that's a problem I don't have. So I breathe. In and out. In and out, while listening to my cousin breathe impatiently through the phone. What I feel in my attempts to conjure up compassion for this woman is pain, actual pain in the center of my chest, like heartburn or the pressure of a finger jabbing me.

And then my daughter enters the room carrying the I-Pod her godfather gave her.

"'Jackson,' let's play 'Jackson!'" she says.

I take the I-Pod from her hand and set it into the speakers. I scroll down to *The Essential Johnny Cash* album and find "Jackson."

That familiar plucking of the guitar begins. I am still breathing, in and out.

"Louder, Mommy, louder!" she says. I watch her lift up her long skirt and tap her foot to the beat.

> *We got married in a fever, hotter than a peppersprout,*
> *We've been talkin' about Jackson, ever since the fire went out.*
> *I'm going to Jackson, I'm gonna mess around,*

Yeah, I'm going' to Jackson,
Look out Jackson town.

Well, go on down to Jackson;
go ahead and wreck your health.
Go play your hand you big talkin' man,
make a big fool of yourself, Yeah, go to Jackson;
go comb your hair!
Honey, I'm gonna snowball Jackson.
See if I care.

"Hello?" my cousin's voice is impatient.

I watch my daughter dance in front of the mirror, twirling, jumping, twisting with her hands on her hips.

"Louder," she yells to me.

I turn the volume up louder. My daughter turns to me and holds out her hands. The pain in my chest is gone. My cousin wants to know what she should tell her kids.

"Tell them the truth," I tell her.

I toss the phone onto the couch and hold my daughter's hands. We dance in circles to June and Johnny Cash's song; never was love and irreverence harmonized as beautifully.

The Theys

Humans respond to rituals profoundly. More persistent loyalty and commitment can be elicited through them than through almost any other means. Taking on a new role in the eyes of the public and witnessing its decisive approval presents the young with a validated reinforcement that gives him or her a feeling of 'belonging' to the new status. The initiate does not play the new role; he or she becomes the role.

"The Lack of Rite of Passage"

Hans Sebald, *Adolescence: A Social Psychological Analysis*

The baby is 31 weeks old now. Norah and I debate how much the baby will weigh at birth; she guesses 8 ½ pounds, I am hoping smaller, for her sake. Presently, the baby weighs 3.5 pounds, and measures about eighteen inches from head to toe. The baby opens and closes its eyes, it is becoming accustomed to the world of light and dark. Its facial muscles strengthen day by day, its face now capable of different expressions.

We attend a birthday party for a friend's son. I stand in the corner watching my daughter interact with the other children; she is a social animal, much more so than me, she is a child who loves a party, a standing-room-only party with loud music and very little fresh air.

Suddenly: *The big day is coming! I am so excited for you!*

The voice is followed by clapping close to my ear. The woman standing next me is an acquaintance, an acquaintance who sends me holiday cards, whose middle name and place of birth I do not know, nor does she know mine, but evidently she does know something about me. The expression on my face is one of genuine surprise; I have no idea what she is talking about. But when I look deeper into her eyes, I know. I am beginning to recognize this gaze: the eyebrows are raised, the pupils enlarged, focused on every angle, every wrinkle, every shadow on my face, assessing, examining, searching for a twitch, a slight nod — some recognition of what she is talking about. Of course I know now the news she is referring to, but I do not let on, not yet. She nods her head, raises her eyebrows higher, but I say nothing. What this is becoming is a test of wills, a stand-off, so to speak: who will give in first? I am hoping she will retreat, that she will read beneath my blank expression to my repulsion of her assumptions, of her claim to the news which I never shared with her, news she has heard from someone, somewhere, news that she has not been granted the privilege to spread. I am hoping that she will read in my face sadness, defeat over the fact that her sudden ownership to my news has opened up a world that I suspected was out there, the world of "them" of "theys" who somehow obtain information and, like a sculpture made of papier maiche, gather bits of this and that and mold it and form it into whatever shape they wish, then pour foul-smelling goop all over it until it is solid, unbreakable, impenetrable as stone.

"Do you know if it's a boy or girl?"

She calls my bluff and breaks the silence. Her smile now like glass, hard, transparent, unmoving.

The few facts that I know about my inquisitor are that she is a mother of four; if her husband simply "looks" at her she becomes pregnant. She feels better pregnant than *not*; and all four births happened naturally (no drugs) with the help of a doula who rubbed some kind of ointment all over her vagina while she was in labor to prevent tearing, and walla! Out slid each baby, and not even one tiny tear. In short, she was built to carry babies, it is her badge of honor. The reason why I know these facts is because she offered them up to another woman ten minutes ago while standing in front of the punch bowl, and I happened to be standing too close to the punch bowl to ignore her.

She is still waiting for my answer.

What I want to ask her is this: Be honest, do you really care whether we are having a boy or a girl? Is our news truly news which evokes applause from you? Be truthful now. You confuse me with your seemingly benign smile and your steadfastness to know, to stand before me and to not back down until you get what you want. Tell me what to do? Tell me how to answer you? I know what my polite upbringing dictates, I know what my father and mother would do if they were standing here in my shoes: they would smile, pull up their boot straps, and take that high road, that terrible road nice people always take, the one unpaved, scattered with potholes and back-breaking hills, lined with dog shit and loud children.

Then again, perhaps I am being unfair.

If I were actually carrying the baby her questioning would be expected. "Certain transitions are universal," the sociologist Hans Sebald writes. "Birth, puberty, assumption of adult responsibility, marriage, parenthood, and death are examples of universal experiences. These and other crises are usually accompanied by rites of passage, designed to carry the individual from one phase of human experience to another." But I have no pregnant belly, and I have not participated in a *rite of passage* signaling to the world my new status as a mother of two because no such rite of passage exists for this situation. "Absence of a transition rite reduces awareness and clarity of one's status and creates maladjustment," Sebald adds. So that is the problem, I am maladjusted, I feel maladjusted, I am suffering from maladjustment; it sounds like a digestive disorder.

I look over at my daughter. She is dancing in the middle of a circle of children. She sticks out her bum and shakes it, waving her arms, full-belly laughing. She does not care that her pants have slid down her hips revealing her purple underpants, or that she is missing a sock. She shakes her head, opens her mouth full of crooked, white teeth and *hoots* like an owl or a train, one cannot be sure which, but she is marvelous.

"We don't know if it's a boy or girl." I deliver my answer ineloquently, I stutter, and the last two words come out sounding like *org-g-gle*. Why is the act of speaking about this, the actual physicality of forming the words with my tongue and lips, so painful?

> Chances are if you enter a surrogacy arrangement you would be the first person everyone you know has ever met who has partaken in a surrogacy agreement. So like it or not, to them, you represent the entire surrogacy experience and community. You may not wish to be the sole representative of surrogacy arrangements to so many people but that's what you would be. Feelings run high when it comes to surrogacy and reproduction in general. Misconceptions are many and chances are you will end up answering the same serious and ridiculous questions over and over again. It's a good idea to be prepared, to plan ahead how you would explain surrogacy to those around you you know well, those whom are acquaintances, and those whom you hardly know at all who insist on sharing their unsolicited opinions. If you think you will be unable to manage defending your choice to others this may be a sign that surrogacy is not right for you.

I read this on the page entitled, "Common Public Thoughts on Surrogacy" on EverythingSurrogacy.com. My first reaction to the tough love of this advice is to laugh, like someone gone mad, then to cry over the pressure of it. I imagine my husband and me spending a Friday night at home role playing: he is the pushy outsider with ridiculous questions about surrogacy and I am me, the ill-prepared coward who suffers from a speech impediment. We take notes, we speak in different accents, we argue (he is not being *ridiculous* enough!); eventually we grow tired and bored and open a bottle of wine. Not only do I wake up the next morning with a terrible hang-over, but I wake up with the realization that I am still the ill-prepared coward, unable to manage defending our choice.

What follows this declaration on page one of EverythingSurrogacy.com is seven pages of quotes from people representing every imaginable stand on the subject. I read the first sentence from the first quote: "I feel so badly for Bill, I don't know how he could let his wife carry some other man's child — " I stop reading and ask myself if I really want to read more. This is one of those moments in life when you have to decide if ignorance is the better choice, and my gut tells me that today it is; just walk away, turn off the computer, and walk away. This moment is reminiscent of a moment in childhood when I came upon Alex Comfort's book, *The Joy Of Sex*, in my father's closet. My mother had thrown my father a surprise party for his 40th birthday and everyone brought gag gifts. I was ten and I remember sitting in the corner of our living room watching my father open his gifts, and listening to the loud laughing that ensued. The theme seemed to be sex and death, and it was difficult for me to keep everything straight between the obscene gifts and the obscene comments, but it was all very fascinating. His cousin Joe gave him a bottle of embalming fluid, the use of which was explained to me later; there were many coffee cups shaped like breasts in all different shapes, sizes and colors, there were a pair of pantyhose with an "extra leg," and dirty books and subscriptions to magazines like *Hustler* and *Playboy*. It was inevitable that I would go searching for these gifts the next day to examine and explore them in the privacy of my own room, and *The Joy of Sex* was the first gift I found. The book from the outside was a safe black and white, much like a text book, and when I fanned the pages quickly in front of my eyes I could see no color, just a blur of a bearded man and woman who appeared to be wrestling; somewhere within my curiosity I was thankful there were no pictures in color. So the moment of truth came: do I hide the book under my shirt and take it to my room? Or do I leave it here in the closet and maintain my safe, ignorant state of mind about bearded men and women?

I took the book to my room.

The shock, the fascination, the horror, the overriding state of bafflement that I felt reading through *The Joy of Sex* is very much the same as today, reading through the quotes on EverythingSurrogacy.com. Like the different positions illustrated in the book (the "Viennese Oyster?"), the opinions expressed in the quotes are opinions that had never occurred to me, in fact, they are opinions I never thought possible. Constance, from Kentucky, believes that "people who can't have children of their own should just accept it as a handicap like any other;" an Anonymous writer believes that "it's sick for a woman to make a child with the intention of giving it away to a stranger and it's even sicker to hire someone like that;" Rick from Texas is tired of everybody playing God, "God should control all life, not doctors and surrogate mothers who need a dollar;" and Jennifer from New York believes that surrogacy is just what impatient people do because they can't wait long enough to adopt a child: "Adoption takes a very long time and these people are fussy about the color of the child...I also hate the argument that all that's left are special needs children. Just because a child is not born in America or isn't white doesn't mean it has special needs. I think it's these parents who insist on having white kids related to them that have the special needs."

The Voice of Reason on EverythingSurrogacy.com, whose voice echoes in my head like that of the Wizard of Oz or my fifth grade religion teacher, Rev. Milly Joyce, follows these opinions with one last bit of sage advice: "The reasons people feel negatively about surrogacy are many. Some arguments are logical and well founded while others are illogical. Before entering a surrogate arrangement you should try to understand the different views people have about surrogacy without being judgmental, just as you wish those around you to listen to your views without judging you."

Here's the truth of the matter: I do not want to imagine the anger and the disgust that motivates Constance from Kentucky and Rick from Texas and Jennifer from New York to take time out of their day to find a website on surrogacy where they can sit before a computer screen and unleash rage. But to not want to imagine this is very much like sitting in my bedroom all those years ago and not wanting to imagine my mother and father in the various positions Comfort illustrates in *The Joy of Sex*. It seems I am re-visiting a lesson I learned as child: what I *want* and what is reality do not always align (after all these years it is still a terrible discovery). Of course age and the practice of denial help to lessen these discrepancies: when I shut the computer off, Constance, Rick, and Jennifer are gone; when I replaced my father's sex book on his closet shelf the strangeness I felt being in the same room as my parents eventually disappeared. But the inevitable face-to-face inquisitions that I have already begun to experience will not be so easily shrugged off because the hot topic is not sex or rage, it's a baby, a baby whose beginnings are simply different, a difference that cannot be changed or ignored or hidden; a difference I have failed time and time again to defend.

I feel as if two worlds are converging into me. There is the world that Norah represents, a world of such selflessness and generosity, a world where strangers offer themselves up in order to help another, and then there is this other world of judgment and cynicism, the fear of anything different. The more they converge the more desperation I feel to keep them apart; the more they converge the more I distrust, the less willing I am to share our good news. By not telling the world how proud I am of Norah and our unborn baby I am, in a sense, giving credence to the cynicism and suspicions. By keeping our news a secret I am not rising above the ignorance. The truth is I am no match against the misconceptions, at least not for today.

I am still at the birthday party. The woman is still standing close to me, her arms crossed, her back to the rest of the room, lest someone try to interrupt. Her inquiries have now moved to logistics: *Are you actually going to be in the room for the delivery? How does all of that work?* She waves her hand in the air, the vague, squiggly, imaginary circles referring to *that. Do you hold the baby first or does your surrogate? How does all of that work?* Her forehead wrinkles, her hand waves, weaving more imaginary circles over our heads. I think of that cheerleader, the one with the sparkling white smile and extra high kicks whom I impersonated so well during my campaign for normalcy, before all of *this* began; I wonder what happened to her. I imagine she was shot, or perhaps she's in rehab somewhere lying quietly by a pool.

I have noticed lately that I am drawn to strangers: the nice lady at the coffee shop around the corner who has a teething nine month old, the waitress at the vegan diner who misses her home state of Texas, the man from Bangladesh who owns the health food store and gives my daughter free candy because his young daughter is in Bangladesh, and he hasn't seen her in two years. I love their stories, their friendliness, I love that they ask nothing about my life. Perhaps this is a cheap form of friendship, friendship that asks nothing, that gives no solutions or advice, that balances just on the surface and disappears with the slightest change of wind; it is human contact with no strings attached, a bit like prostitution.

Tomorrow my husband and I fly to Indianapolis for Norah's 32-week ultrasound; we will also meet with the lawyer who will have news of our plea for parental rights. I tuck my daughter into bed and tell her that we will be gone in the morning when she wakes up.

"Where are you going?" She asks. I pause, stalling.

"We're going on a plane," I tell her.

"To the beach?" She demands. There is a slight panic in her voice, it has been a cold winter in New York. She has worn her bathing suit around the apartment every day after school, pining away for sun and surf.

"No, we're not going to the beach. We're going to see the baby."

She opens her mouth to say something, then she smiles guiltily and covers her face with the blanket.

"What is it?" I ask.

Without removing the blanket she points her finger to beneath her bed. I reach my hand underneath her bed and feel something. It is a book, a book whose shape and thickness of about 300 pages I know well. I pull Erikson's book out and hold it to my chest. I pull the blanket off her face. She is still smiling.

"Thanks for the book. You will be a good girl tomorrow, yes?"

I can see her mind jumping from thought to thought, then: "The April baby's coming," she whispers, her voice ominous, certain.

I nod my head, yes, it is coming.

Unique Beginnings

The unnaturalness of not knowing your origins makes you feel unnatural. There is the presumption that something is wrong because it can't be told. And when a child is raised with secrets, he feels his whole life to be wrong.

Betty Jean Lifton, *Journey of the Adopted Self*

In Sue Erikson Bloland's book, *In the Shadow of Fame: A Memoir by the Daughter of Erik H. Erikson*, Bloland writes of the secret that plagued her famous father's life from the age of eight: the identity of his biological father. Born in Frankfurt, Germany in 1902, Erikson lived his first three years with his unwed mother, Karla, a woman whose husband, Valdemar Salomonsen, had abandoned her four years before Erikson's conception. Though the name "Salomonsen" appeared on Erikson's birth certificate, this was only a means to cover up his illegitimacy. Four months after Erikson's birth, Valdemar's father provided Karla with proof that his son had died, leaving Karla widowed, thus free to marry. Then in 1905 Karla married Theodor Homburger, a well-respected pediatrician whom Erikson was told was his real father.

It is at the age of eight, after a strange conversation with an old peasant woman who asks the young Erikson, "Do you know who your father is?" that Erikson confronts his mother; she reveals to him only part of the truth. She admits that Theodor was not his real father and that she had been previously married, leading her son to believe that Valdemar Salomonsen was Erikson's father.

Erikson later wrote:

> All through my earlier childhood, they kept secret from me the fact that my mother had been married previously; that I was the son of a Dane who had abandoned her before my birth. They apparently thought that such secretiveness was not only workable (because children then were not held to know what they had not been told) but advisable, so that I would feel thoroughly at home in their home. As children will do, I played in with this and more or less forgot the period before the age of 3, when Mother and I had lived alone.

What stands out in this passage, written when Erikson was in his seventies, is how Erikson seems to imply that the "Dane" was his mother's first husband, which was not the case. "Even in his old age it was still a source of shame to this celebrated man that he had been an illegitimate child," Bloland writes.

Throughout his life Erikson's mother, Karla, would not discuss this "Dane," the man whom, for reasons unknown, could not or would not marry her. Karla claimed that she had promised Theodor "lifelong secrecy and she wished to remain faithful to her commitment." Even when confronted by Erikson's wife, Joan, who simply wanted information about their children's genetic history, Karla refused to discuss Erikson's biological father. Bloland writes:

> I have heard this story many times over the years and have always felt angry with my grandmother for what seems an incomprehensible lack of empathy with my father's need to identify his missing father. I struggle to respect her commitment to Theodor as well as the demands of her own pride, which was, after all, twice damaged.

"Adoption was the great theme of Erikson's life," Erikson's boyhood friend Peter Blos told Betty Lifton. "He talked about it all the time, speculated on the possibilities." Sadly, Erikson never learned the truth, he never learned the identity of his biological father. When Betty Lifton asked Erikson why he did not pursue the identity of his father more "vigorously," Erikson replied: "If my father hadn't cared enough about me to want me then, why should I look him up now?"

It is startling for me to read Erikson's reply to Lifton; it is startling to feel his defensiveness, his disguised indifference — all failed attempts to cover up his hurt. It is startling because Erikson, one of the most influential psychological thinkers of the 20th century, is acting, playing the invincible son, the son who hides behind a brave front. He is pretending not to feel what he so obviously feels. In Bloland's opinion, her father's reluctance to pursue his biological father is two-fold: to protect himself from further heartbreak (perhaps his father never wanted to know him), and to protect his mother from a truth that had caused her so much pain.

For weeks I think about Erikson's mother and her young son. I think about the year 1902, the year of Erikson's birth, and the shame, estrangement, and even dangers that would have surrounded a pregnant, unwed woman, in my attempts to understand why a mother would withhold such an important truth from her child.

And then I look at myself and I understand.

I am beginning to understand the temptation of re-writing history, of re-creating that which you desire for your child, that which would be acceptable, uncontroversial, safe. How much easier it would have been for Karla and for Erikson had Valdemar Salomonsen been Erikson's biological father — or even better, Theodor, the respected pediatrician.

How much easier it would have been if I had not suffered complications after my daughter's birth, if my placenta had simply slipped out of my body like it was supposed to; how much easier it would have been for this second child of ours to be growing inside my body, here in New York, instead of inside another woman's in Indiana.

Like Karla and Erikson, I am hiding from the truth, toying with the possibilities of somehow changing it, hiding it, perhaps disregarding it altogether.

***

In Betty Lifton's book, *Journey of the Adopted Self*, she explores through her own experience as an adopted child, as well as countless other adults who have been adopted, the world of the adopted person and the adopted person's quest to find a sense of self. Lifton writes of the moment she learned she was adopted:

> I didn't realize that, like Peter [Pan], I wasn't exactly human until I was seven years old. It was the moment my mother told me I was adopted. Like most adoptive parents faced with breaking such bleak news, she tried to make adoption sound special, but I could feel the penetrating chill of its message. I was not really her child. I had come from somewhere else, a place shrouded in mystery…As I listened, I could feel a part of myself being pulled into the darkness of that mystery—a place already carved out by Peter and the lost children. I would never be the same again.

I want to understand why the good intentions of wanting a child, a want motivated, presumably, by love so often results in irredeemable pain. Lifton's description of how alone and changed she felt at seven-years-old carries with it the gravity and permanence of death; for her, the repercussions of adoption seem to be without hope, without redemption, at only seven the story of childhood has ended unhappily, and the intimation of the next phase of life is one plagued with unanswered questions, unresolved conflicts, in essence, a life stuck. After her mother breaks the news, she tells her daughter that this was to be their secret: "Hers and mine," Lifton remembers. "I was not to share it with anyone—not even my father. It would break his heart if he suspected I knew." I read this memory of Lifton's as if I am reading a scene from a Shakespeare play (the moment before

Othello kills Desdemona, the seconds before Romeo takes his own life); with each word Lifton uses to describe her and her mother's secret pact, I can feel what a terrible mistake her mother has made, I can feel how damaging and irreversible the consequences will be.

The question of one's beginnings takes me back two years to the office of the Center for Surrogate Parenting to the question posed by the counselor, the same question on the questionnaire that my husband and I so quickly skipped over on the car ride to Annapolis, the question, like the possibility of another child that seemed so unreal that day, perhaps even impossible, grows more real to me now as the days pass. And if that question alone wasn't complex enough, I now have a question of my own: How will this unborn child feel when he or she looks at our daughter, the first born, the older sibling: how will he or she feel upon learning that I carried her? How will he or she feel when the truth is revealed that our first born, who loves to hear stories of my cravings for scrambled eggs while she was in my tummy, need never worry about such a concept as "unique beginnings?" Have our good intentions—the desire for another child, the desire for our daughter to share a life with a sibling, and for that sibling to share a life with her—which could only be realized with the help of a surrogate, placed this unborn child in an inescapably strange place? Will he or she feel like 7-year-old Lifton felt, pulled into darkness, stuck in a mysterious place with no escape? At the beginning of Lifton's book she quotes James Barrie's *Peter Pan in Kensington Gardens:*

> "Then I shan't be exactly human?" Peter asked.
> "No."
> "What shall I be?"
> "You will be Betwixt-and-Between," Solomon said, and certainly he was a wise old fellow, for that is exactly how it turned out.

Lifton acknowledges that many people find themselves in this state of "Betwixt and Between," but for her, when her mother told her the truth of her beginnings, this state of ambiguity took on new meaning: "I had come from somewhere else, a place shrouded in mystery, a place that, like myself, was Betwixt and Between."

And here it is again, the ominous sense of doom in imagining the possibility of passing on such a heavy weight to a child. What I feel is perhaps similar to what Lifton's mother must have felt: the wish for the truth to be different.

Assisted reproductive technology and its advances have helped deliver more than 3 million babies into the world since 1978, and the numbers continue to grow. Thus the question of one's unique beginnings and its increasing relevance in our world, in society, continues to grow as well. With the whole array of "unique beginnings" ranging from surrogacy to sperm donors, egg donors to embryo donors, I find that I am not the only one haunted by this question. I search for advice from parents who have already faced that complicated question; I do not find any information on this topic in the surrogacy agency's literature, so I look on the internet. In an article from the BBC News, written in 2001, nine out of ten parents whose children were conceived using donor sperm had not told their children the truth about their unique beginnings. Many of the parents said they had no intention of ever telling their children the truth; and half expressed fear over how such news would effect their 10 to 12-year-olds. In an article entitled, "Surrogacy: The Experience of Commissioning Couples," in *Human Reproduction*, a journal published by the Oxford University Press, 42 couples with a 1-year-old child, born with the help of surrogates, were assessed and interviewed. What the studies found was that all of the couples had told family and friends about the surrogate and had every intention of telling the child in the future. But these were findings from just 42 couples; upon studying further couples the notion of secrecy grew more complex. "The continuation of contact between the family and the surrogate mother will depend on whether the commissioning couples intend to disclose the facts of the surrogacy arrangement to the child," the article states. "Studies of families created by gamete donation have found that the large majority of parents do not intend to disclose the method of conception to the child." The article goes on to site studies that secrecy, about whichever conception method one uses to have a child, would "damage family relationships with a consequent negative impact on the child's psychological development."

And then I find the website I have been looking for: artparenting.org, a website developed by the Harvard Medical School Center for Mental Health and Media, created for parents and children who have been affected by assisted reproductive technology. I learn that the notion of secrecy is not new. The website gives an ART timeline beginning in 1790 when the first successful case of human artificial insemination is performed by the Scottish surgeon John Hunter. "Using simple techniques learned from animal husbandry, small town doctors were able to help their male patients become fathers through artificial insemination. Nobody needed to know that a sperm donor was involved, the doctors reasoned, and the patients were cautioned never to reveal the secret to anyone—especially not the child." Of course today this strategy is criticized. "Secrets can strain family relationships and cause psychological harm to children. They argue that being open with children about their genetic origins lessens any sense of negativity or shame, and protects kids from finding out accidentally in life."

The first example the website gives is of the Gilbert family who finally disclosed their secret to their children when they were twenty-one. Gary battled testicular cancer when he was young, which left him infertile; he and his wife had their twins using a sperm donor. I listen to the audio of the father, Gary:

> I felt I was relieving myself of the biggest load I had carried my entire life. I felt that because I wanted them to know—and I wanted them to know before I wasn't here to tell them myself... now when I told them—I'm crying, Emily's crying, Andrew put his head down on the table and cried. And Emily got on my lap and said, "Dad, it must have been so hard for you to carry this all those years." I would have told them when they were three or four years old...I would have said, "Daddy didn't have enough seeds to make

> mommy pregnant, so we went to the hospital and we borrowed some seeds." As they grew up and had questions about it, I would have addressed it absolutely honestly.

Gary's voice is kind, the love for his kids, his struggle to do the right thing is apparent, as is the love his daughter Emily feels for him as she recounts the moment her dad told her the truth:

> When I was younger, I swore there was this secret. There was this tension between my mom and my dad…I used to ask her, I was like, Mom, what is the secret? There is a secret, I know there's a secret…I was 21, and I was back from school. It was my senior year at UC Santa Barbara…My dad — he just came walking down the stairs kind of sheepishly and he was like, 'Andrew, Emily I want to talk to you." And I just knew that it was something serious…and so we went upstairs into the family kitchen and I sat across from my dad at the table. And my brother was sitting next to me. And I think my mom was standing behind us…because my mom didn't want to have any part in this…my mom was against us knowing the truth because she thought we would never feel like we have these Gilbert genes.

And when her father tells Emily and her brother the truth, Emily describes how her mind is at first focused on his cancer and the fear it had come back — the detail of her and her brother not being related to their father genetically did not occur to her initially. But when she does realize what her father is telling her it is a shock: "I was like, wait a minute! So we're not genetically related to you. This is weird. Like, I just started to cry because I felt bad. It was like, 'Oh my goodness, this is huge!'"

The audio ends there. I would like to know more.

Did the truth change how Emily felt about her father, about herself? My instinct tells me, no; or at least not in a detrimental way. Listening to Gary's audio again, and then to Emily's, the love they feel for each other overrides the story. It is the tone of their voices, their openness, especially Emily's forthrightness and confidence that resonates.

The next example on the website is a family who used surrogacy to have their two children. I recognize the woman's name, Fay Johnson. She is the coordinator of the Center for Surrogate Parenting in the Beverly Hills office. Before reading her story I knew nothing about her except that she had a lovely voice and might have been the nicest person I had ever spoken with over the phone. I listen to her familiar voice on the audio as she explains that she is a DES baby (while her mother was pregnant she was given diethylstilbestrol to prevent miscarriage, which caused uterus malformations, one of the side effects of the DES). She and her late husband used traditional surrogacy to have their two children, Lily and Chase; the surrogate's eggs were used along with Fay's husband's sperm. Fay explains:

> When I first became involved in surrogacy, I really asked myself what was I going to stand for in this? I was one of the first people, and I'd never met another person who had done it. All the way through Lily's birth, I had not met another person who had done it. There is power in truth. So taking that position, I realized I needed to start it when they were infants.

Fay told Lily, her first-born, the story of her unique beginning when she was just six-weeks old. "I really felt if I became comfortable telling the story to her, then when she was old enough to ask questions about it, I would probably be comfortable enough to be able to answer them and completely convince her that I was completely sure of myself." When Lily was 9-years old she told her mom, "Mom, I have it figured out, I am not from your egg!" The revelation occurred when her father had been diagnosed with cancer, when fear and uncertainty had entered their lives. Lily feared that if her father died perhaps she would be sent away to live with the surrogate, the woman whose egg had helped make Lily. Fay responded to Lily's fears by showing her her birth certificate.

> 'See the line where it says mother? That's me. And I am your mother forever. No matter what happens to dad, no one can ever take you from me. I am your mother forever.' And I think that is what she needed to hear.

And then there is 14-year-old Lily's response to her unique beginnings:

> I think it was really good that she told us right off the bat. Because if she hadn't told us, if she were to just tell us when we were 10 or 11 or something, it'd be like, 'So, who's my real mother?' I don't think I'd ever forgive her if she didn't tell me right off the bat. That's just like lying to you for your whole life.

***

In Lawrence J. Friedman's biography of Erik H. Erikson, *Identity's Architect*, Friedman describes a meeting with Erikson in June of 1993, Erikson was about to turn 91 years old. Friedman had been in Copenhagen visiting Erikson's relatives, searching family records, documents, anywhere he could to gather information on the identity of Erikson's biological father. "I was determined to bring him a special birthday gift," Friedman writes. What Friedman brings to Erikson, who sat in a wheelchair in his home in Cambridge, Massachusetts, is a family tree extending from the 18th century, a photograph of Erikson's mother, Karla, as a young woman, and information on two Danish men who might have been Erikson's biological father; the wish to bring Erikson the final gift of his father's identity unfortunately would not come to be.

Friedman describes how Erikson glanced over the family history and the names of the two Danes with "little interest." "I realized," Friedman writes, "that his lifelong quest to discover the identity of his father would remain unfulfilled." But then Friedman watched as Erikson picked up the photograph of his mother and stared down at it.

"What a beauty," Erikson said.

> Although he was very frail and nearly immobile, his eyes had come alive. A smile crossed his face. Erikson was enjoying himself amid the flow of memories of his Danish mother. He glanced at the small Danish flag on the mantel above his fireplace and back again at the photograph.

If ever there was a question about the importance of the truth of our beginnings, of our family history, of the place from where we come, this memory of Erikson at the end of his life, holding an old photograph of his mother in his hands, lays that question to rest.

Dream

I wake up in the middle of the night with my hand pressed against my stomach, surprised to find that I am not carrying a baby. The dream felt so real, the fist moving beneath the skin, the hard shape of you pressed against me, that familiar fluttering. I watched as you sat up, fully upright, your eyes two almonds, staring at me, taking me in, and with a firm kick flipped yourself over, your head, an oval globe, now facing downward toward my pubic bone, your feet pressing against my ribs, showing me your strength as if to say, *Look, mama, I can do it myself.*

And isn't that what I want, for you ultimately not to need me?

March 2nd. I sit on the plane next to the window. It is almost eight in the morning, I watch snow fall onto the wing. We received good news yesterday from our lawyer. The Commissioner for the paternity court in Marion County, Indiana has agreed to issue an order of maternity and paternity, based on the documents filed by our lawyer. The baby's birth certificate will bear my name, not Norah's, thus a hearing will not be required. We will not need to travel back to Indianapolis after the baby's birth for any future court proceedings or undertake any legal procedures in New York.

Our lawyer delivers this news to me with the voice of a champion: we got lucky, she reiterates, reminding me of the Steve Litz case and how Indiana courts are no longer surrogacy-friendly. We got *very* lucky, she says again. I think she was expecting a more dramatic response from me, tears, a joyful scream, perhaps. So I dig deep and give her what she wants: I gush through the phone with gratitude. I hang up the phone. I am grateful, of course, but the baby is ours, it should bear our name.

We are traveling to Indianapolis for the 32-week ultrasound, and to meet Norah's doctor. He has delivered all of Norah's children, her own as well as the other two children she carried for other families. During the two-hour flight I feel sullen and tired. My husband looks up from his paper and asks me what's wrong. *I feel sullen and tired,* I tell him. He lays his hand on my head for a few seconds, then goes back to his paper. I turn away and stare out the window. It is a wonderful gift to not always have to explain oneself.

When I see Norah standing in front of the hospital it feels like crossing over into a different world, like walking off an airplane into a foreign place where the sounds and smells and quality of air is different. As I step out of the car I feel my two selves separate. This moment of separation is not metaphorical it is literal, physical in the sudden change of my breathing, now even, in my posture, now straight, in my head, now held high; I feel lighter, the dark mood swirling around me has been replaced with something lighter, something that feels a bit like happiness as I walk toward Norah.

And the other self? The one who suffers from confusion and self-pity, shame and cowardice? She sits in the rental car sulking, with the windows up.

Before the doctor's appointment we go to lunch. My husband parks the car and Norah and I stand inside the restaurant waiting for a table. She wears a white maternity blouse, the small pleats gather along the top of her belly; she carries the baby high, and her tummy protrudes out, from behind she does not look pregnant. Her skin glows and her green eyes look blue today; she is lovely.

Over the course of lunch she tells us that people have begun to notice that she is pregnant, so naturally questions follow. I smile and nod, unable to comment, afraid she will see through me, right into my own fear of such questions and my attempts to escape when confronted with them. She tells us about a nice old man who works in her office building who congratulated her on her pregnancy, then he asked where her wedding ring was. I feel my hands begin to sweat and my foot begin to tap on the floor, imagining how I would escape such a question, but Norah just smiles and shakes her head. She told the old man she didn't have a wedding ring, and wasn't planning on getting one any time soon, which left him speechless. He wished her luck, and that was the end of it.

I study her expression, her amusement; she is genuinely unaffected by all of it. She is brave, unapologetic, serene. As she sits across from me, I pray she does not ask me what I have told people, I don't want her to know that nice, nosy, old men terrify me. Here she is, carrying our baby, and yet I cannot find the courage to hold my head high and face ridiculous questions; it seems such a small thing, what has been asked of me, and yet I continue to hide from it.

My husband has not seen the baby since the 6-week ultrasound back in September. The ultrasound screen is located high on the wall, almost to the ceiling, it is slanted downward. Norah lies on the table and my husband and I stand side by side a few feet away from her staring up at the screen. The baby has been breech for a few weeks now, and we have been hoping that it will turn head down so that a Cesarean section will not be needed. When the nurse switches the screen on we see something dart across it, quick, elusive like a fish behind the glass of an aquarium. The four of us gasp—Ah! Where did it go? Oh, wait there it is! Norah comments that the baby is rarely still, and it is true, the baby will not lie still long enough to allow us a good look at it, and that's why we are here, to actually see it, to get acquainted with this baby that has seemed more like a dream or an idea than our actual child.

The nurse fears she will not be able to get a good picture if the baby doesn't stop moving. Minutes pass—then suddenly the baby falls asleep. Its head is slumped to the side, the hands folded beneath the chin. The nurse tells us that the baby is no longer breech, its head is down, exactly where it should be. I watch the baby sleep. The screen reminds me of the small black and white television set we used to have in our kitchen growing up that never gave a clear picture. The baby's face is small, delicate, shaped like an egg, its nose like a triangle, the mouth parted like my daughter's when she is in a deep sleep. I stand here, staring up at the screen and I feel both love and detachment; and I do not know how this is possible. My husband squeezes my arm, he cannot stop smiling and pointing and questioning the nurse to be sure that he has spotted the correct body parts. He is just as he was when he witnessed ultrasounds with our daughter, the gleeful spectator, the beaming father. He wraps his arm around my neck and pulls me to him. *Can you believe it?* He asks me. *Can you believe it?*

The three of us sit side by side in the waiting room of Norah's doctor's office and I feel people stare, sizing us up, wondering about the dynamics of this strange threesome (clearly, Norah is not our daughter). We do not have to wait long, the nurse escorts us into the examining room and my husband and I sit in the corner, Norah sits up on the table, and we wait. The doctor enters the room. He is friendly with a warm smile and an obvious fondness for Norah. He takes her blood pressure, she tells him she is short of breath and he tells her that is normal, and then we chat. He has done his homework on us, on my medical history, but he seems most fascinated by the fact that we live in New York City; he has been to New York a few times, and every time he can't wait to leave, he doesn't care much for city living. He assures us of Norah's good health, of the health of our baby, and speculates that Norah will be induced in the 37th or 38th week, though we will have to wait and see for a definitive date. Before he leaves he adds one last thing: he tells us how lucky we are to have Norah helping us. Then he looks at Norah and shakes his head: *She is an amazing woman*, he adds. I nearly jump out of my chair to prove to him how much we agree with him, how grateful we are for her. *We are so grateful for her*, I tell him, *so grateful!* I understand the importance of the doctor's statement to Norah, sitting by herself on the examining table, her body enduring another pregnancy, preparing for another birth; I understand how important it is for her to feel his support. It is because of Norah that I ignore what felt a bit like condescension in his reminder to us of what we inherently know and feel, like a parent reminding his child to say 'thank you.' I follow him to the door, repeating how much we adore Norah, how much we appreciate everything she has done for us, how special she is; I want him to believe me. He smiles, nods, shakes my hand, then my husband's hand, then he leaves; and I'm not sure he believed me.

At the lawyer's office in downtown Indianapolis we are scheduled to sign court documents in the presence of a notary, documents which will ensure the proper birth certificate when the baby is born. It is an hour of signing and awkward chit-chat in a conference room adorned with life-size portraits of former law partners, white men with grim expressions, wearing conservative, dark suits posing next to chairs, desks, and fireplaces. The chit-chat takes on a life of its own as yet another secretary joins us with more papers and more commentary; perhaps the lawyer and her staff are trying to make us more comfortable by sharing with us the names of their children, stories of their latest surgeries, and facts about tornadoes. I nod, I smile, I try to act interested, but I feel as if my eyeballs might fall out of my head, or I may begin to drool. At one point my husband and I glance at each other and begin to laugh silently, and I have to leave the room to compose myself. This is not a proud moment. It has been a long day. When I return the lawyer gives us a bowl of stale candy and the three of us empty the bowl.

We are late for our flight. My husband is calm, he likes the challenge of arriving at the airport five minutes before the plane takes off, but I am on edge. I hurry toward security, with my bag, driver's license and ticket in hand, leaving my husband behind; I cannot miss this plane. Then something hits my foot, and I feel myself trip and then — oh, God, fall hard to the ground, the strap of my bag twisted around my leg. Because I am in Indiana, arguably home to some of the nicest people on the planet, a crowd descends, circling around me offering help. *I'm fine, I'm fine, thank you*, I tell them, waving them away. As people begin to gather the contents of my bag that are strewn all over the floor I implore them to please stop, *I am fine, please, I am fine*. But no one listens to me, no one is backing off. Then I feel a hand on my arm and I shake it away. I am fine! *I don't need your help!* The hand was my husband's. *I don't need your help*, I tell him again as I pull myself up. *I don't need anybody's help*. I watch the nice people gathered around me begin to back away, realizing they are in the presence of a possible marital dispute. I pick up the rest of my things and stuff them in my bag.

We make our flight, and I sit next to the window staring out at the dark sky. I don't speak to my husband during the two-hour flight for no other reason than I have no one else to ignore.

On the way home from the airport I begin to feel guilty. I have ruined a day that should have ended in celebration: the baby is healthy, it is no longer breech; Norah is healthy; the baby's birth certificate will bear my name; on every count it was a successful day. Sitting in the back seat of the taxi, I feel my two selves merge together again, at once at odds, though strangely bonded in this uncomfortable state of unease that has been our home for the last nine months. I rub my left knee.

"Does your knee hurt?" My husband asks.

"No, it doesn't hurt." I remove my hand from my knee, turning away from him, and stare out the window.

My knee is killing me. I want to keep rubbing it, to numb the pain a bit, but I'd rather feel the pain than admit to it. As we cross the Triboro Bridge and drive into Manhattan I feel the hot stubbornness of me, it races through my veins, pulses in the center of my knee. This is who I am. It has taken me thirty-five years to understand that I am a person who hates asking for help, because in order to ask for help one must admit to defeat, and defeat occurs when one's shortcomings come to light. This day has been, on the one hand, miraculous: when I kissed Norah goodbye I felt love for her, standing before me, large-bellied and glowing, she has challenged my skeptical view of the world and proven that goodness remains. But this day has also been a nightmare, every part of today was defined by my inability, as if I were wearing a sign on my back announcing my inability to do anything useful. It feels as if I have been thrust from my once private and rather solitary existence into a commune, where I am forced to share my life with strangers, to not only live amicably and dependently among them, but gratefully as well. How am I to endure this? Why does asking for help feel more like drowning than being saved?

During the five weeks I spent in the hospital on bed rest, pregnant with my daughter, friends and family would call and say, "It must be so awful for you, to be just sitting there day after day; not to mention the food." But the truth was, it wasn't awful at all, in a strange way I liked it, and the food wasn't bad.

"Freud was once asked what he thought a normal person should be able to do well," Erik H. Erikson writes in *Identity: Youth and Crisis*.

> The questioner probably expected a complicated, "deep" answer. But Freud simply said, "*Lieben und arbeiten*" ("to love and to work"). It pays to ponder on this simple formula; it grows deeper as you think about it. For when Freud said "love," he meant the generosity of intimacy as well as genital love; when he said love and work, he meant a general productiveness which would not preoccupy
> the individual to the extent that he might lose his right or capacity to be a sexual and a loving being.

Though I was ordered by my doctors to do nothing but lie in bed and try not to move, and though they explained that early labor would most likely occur, despite my best efforts to stay still, I felt empowered by the job I had to do: my daughter's life depended on my best efforts to stop my amniotic fluid from leaking, and to thereby stop the labor and delivery of a 32-week-old fetus. Sitting in that hospital bed day after day was not awful at all, it was work, in the most productive and rewarding sense; I felt useful to my unborn daughter, to my husband, I felt as if I had a purpose. "To love and to work," I can think of no better reasons to live.

But with this second child, what work have I done? How have I shown my love? Surrogacy, is without question, a miracle in reproductive technology, from a physiological standpoint it offers options to women with reproductive limitations, this is unarguable, but as miraculous and as generous as it is, the technology, for me, has clashed with the psychological aspect of the natural order of things, of our natural life cycles that I had never realized were so ingrained in my consciousness. Surrogacy turns the absolutism of carrying a child, of childbirth itself, upside down, the same way a child dying before its parents throws off the natural order. It feels as if I am part of an actual transition in human evolution where the rules of reproduction are changing drastically. This is not a judgment or a vilification of surrogacy, this has nothing to do with jealousy or resentment of women who choose to be surrogates, this is biological bewilderment, imbued with feelings of idleness and futility. To be a woman and to take on the role of bystander to the ever-changing human functions of conception, growth, and birth, all of which nature has bequeathed solely to women, seems to me a precarious state of being. And yet, I suppose it is important to consider this question: why nature chose women for the job in the first place? In my unscientific opinion the answer seems obvious, because women have the makeup to handle it. Perhaps the resolution I seek lies here, in a woman's inherent strength to overcome, to stand up, and to keep moving.

***

At the end of David McCullough's biography, *John Adams*, he writes about the president's remaining years (he lived to almost 91), filled with family and visits from friends and a continued love of reading, letter-writing, and work. In letters written to his old friend, Benjamin Rush, Adams describes his work days, which typically began at five or six in the morning, feeding his cattle, working in his hayfield, "pottering" among his fruit trees and vegetable garden, and building stone walls:

> I call for my leavers and iron bars, for my chisels, drills and wedges to split rocks, and for my wagon to cart seaweed for manure upon my farm. I mount my horse and ride on the seashore, and I walk upon Mount Wollaston and Stoneyfield Hill.

McCullough writes of the importance to Adams of

joining in the actual physical labor of his farm, of maintaining the companionship with the workers with whom he had known and worked for years. "Stoneyfield was no gentleman's farm and he [Adams] no gentleman farmer. The farm that had sustained the Adamses and their family through the lean years of the Revolution would have to sustain them again. They could expect no additional income."

When my husband reads this sudden diversion into the life of John Adams, he will no doubt shake his head, though he will not be surprised. I "discovered" John Adams soon after my daughter's birth and have since read everything I can get my hands on about him. McCullough's biography sits permanently on my bedside table next to a photo of my husband and daughter; I have adopted the old Massachusett as a member of my family. To say that I am enamored with John Adams, a portly, balding man who described himself as "looking rather like a short, thick Archbishop of Canterbury," and who would eventually lose all of his teeth, would not be an exaggeration, because the mind (and Adams's mind was still sharp upon his death) is undeniably alluring, and I find myself inexorably drawn to him. Strong-willed, brilliant, fiery, stubborn, a man who not only read voraciously every one of the 3,000 books in his private library, but actually argued and debated the authors in the margins of these books with his own notes and rebuttals. Adams read such writers as Cicero and Tacitus in Latin, and Plato and Thucydides in Greek; he read all of Shakespeare twice, loved English poetry, and treated the few women authors, in particular Mary Wollstonecraft, with the same attention and zeal. Adams preferred to read books written by people whose philosophies he disagreed with in order to satisfy his drive and his need to exercise the mind.

"The only question remaining with me," Adams wrote to Cotton Tufts after his defeat to Jefferson for a second term, "is what shall I do with myself? Something I must do, or ennui will rain upon me in buckets." He was a great orator and debater, and over the years when Congress was on break and later, when he lost the presidency and was forced into retirement, reading late into the night and arguing with dead writers kept him busy, sharp, and exhilarated. "He was blessed with great courage and good humor," McCullough writes, "yet subject to spells of despair, and especially when separated from his family or during periods of prolonged inactivity." Work was what made Adams tick, it made him feel useful, it made him feel as if he had a purpose. A man like Adams could not enjoy or feel pride for the stone wall surrounding Stoneyfield Farm if he had not had a hand in building it.

So how does my life align with a president's who has been dead for 180 years? I suppose it is the obvious answer: that human nature has not changed, and there is comfort to be found in witnessing a man who could not bear idleness, a great man who battled himself and what he believed to be shortcomings for much of his life, finally attain some peace.

> [Adams] had himself, he told Rush, an 'immense load of errors, weaknesses, follies and sins to mourn over and repent of.' These were 'the only affliction' of his present life. But St. Paul had taught him to rejoice ever more and be content.
> 'This phrase *rejoice ever more* shall never be out of my heart, memory or mouth again as long as I live, if I can help it. This is my perfectibility of man.'

To live and to work, to rejoice and to be content. These are the ingredients of a life being fully lived; they wipe away the self-pity, the despair, they seem to whisper: get on with it now.

Birth Story

As soon as we're born, we're dead. Our birth
and our death are just one thing. It's like the tree:
when there's a root, there must be twigs. When
there are twigs, there must be a root. You can't
have one without the other. It's a little funny to
see how at a death people are so grief-stricken
and distracted, fearful and sad, and at a birth
how happy and delighted. It's delusion; nobody
has ever looked at it clearly. I think if you really
want to cry, then it would be better to do so when
someone's born. For actually birth is death, death
is birth, the root is the twig, the twig is the root. If
you've got to cry, cry at the root, cry at the birth.
Look closely: if there was no birth, there would
be no death. Can you understand this?

Ajahn Chah, "Our Real Home"

But, honestly, how can we really look at birth in that light?
The moment when the head passes safely through the birth canal
and the cry cuts through the silence of the room, how can we not
cry and laugh out of joy? Out of pure amazement and wonder that
a life exists, that in spite of everything it lives.

In the beginning of his book, *On Fertile Ground*, the
anthropologist Peter T. Ellison, writes of a night in 1984 when he
and his wife are preparing dinner in the Ituri, a tropical rain forest
located in the Ituri region of eastern Democratic Republic of the
Congo. Suddenly Ellison's research assistant, Kazimiri, a Lese
villager, appears on the road. Kazimiri has come because his wife,

Elena, who is only seven months pregnant, is in labor. Earlier in the day nuns from the south had visited the village delivering medicines, and after examining Elena had expressed concern over how low she was carrying. Kazimiri asks Ellison if he can use their truck to drive Elena to the mission for medical care; by foot it would take two days, by truck five or six hours, at least. Ellison and his research team agree to help. As they drive the truck toward the village to pick up Elena, they hear voices calling out to them. When Ellison asks Baudoin, another villager accompanying them, what the voices are saying, Baudoin tells them that the birth has already happened, twin boys. Ellison writes,

> Soon two of the women appeared in the door of the hut to display the babies. They were tiny and shriveled, frailer than any healthy newborn. One was clearly dead, but the woman holding him jiggled his limp limbs and made the tiny head rock unnaturally back and forth. The other infant breathed weakly and made tiny movements of his own. They were soon taken back inside. I glimpsed Elena sitting in a corner of the hut with her back against a post, a piece of cloth draped loosely around her body, her hands motionless in her lap, her face blank.

Fast forward a year later, when Ellison and his wife are in the birthing room of a hospital in Boston, awaiting the birth of their first child. It has been more than twenty-four hours and the birth is not progressing; forceps have been tried without success, the baby's head cannot make it through the birth canal, so a Caesarean section is the only option. And a few minutes later a healthy son is born.

Until I had my daughter three and a half years ago, no one had ever spoken to me about the dangers of childbirth. Death in childbirth seemed to me a tragedy of the distant past, like the plague or leprosy; because of modern medicine, I believed those things just didn't happen anymore. I had always taken for granted a healthy birth. But of course I was wrong. In the U.S. the maternal mortality rate is approximately 7.7 deaths per 100,000 pregnancies; but you never hear about them in the news. According to estimates developed by the World Health Organization and UNICEF, in the year 2000 the number of maternal deaths for the world was 529,000. These deaths were almost equally divided between Africa (251,000), and Asia (253,000), with about 4% (22,000) occurring in Latin America and the Caribbean, and less than 1% (2,500) in more developed regions of the world.

I have thought often about Elena, far away in Africa — was she able to have more children? Did they survive? Did she survive? And I think of Ellison and his wife, witnesses to two completely different birth stories, and how this experience changed them. "Both of these stories point to another story, the story of the shaping of human procreation," Ellison begins.

> Both point to the hazards inherent in reproduction itself, the risk of death that shadows new life. Both point to constraints that must be accommodated: the physical difficulty of passing a full-term head through a female pelvis, the difficulty of growing two fetuses to full term. Both whisper of the pitiless process of natural selection that has shaped all features of our biology, reproduction included.

Throughout his book Ellison weaves together the history of reproductive biology with the human experience, two forces that sometimes clash, like with Elena whose second twin ultimately died; while at other times the two co-exist peaceably, like with Ellison's own son who lived and is now a teenager. "Dramas like this," Ellison writes, "repeated countless billions of times in our evolutionary history, have endowed us with our physiological capacities and limitations and shape us still."

Our lives seem to exist in a constant balance between these capacities and limitations, very much like a vaginal birth, where the outcome depends on the relationship between two things: the size of the baby's head and the diameter of the mother's pelvis. When I share with my husband Ellison's analogy that the passing of a full-term head through a woman's pelvis is very much like swallowing a baseball, his face loses color; he had no idea. What is even more astounding to me is how late in pregnancy, hormones are released in order to "loosen the ligaments" that join the two halves of the pelvis together so that during delivery these ligaments may stretch a bit in order to widen the diameter of the pelvis, thereby helping to make room for the passing of the baby's head. How incredible the body is in its physiological ability to adapt, to bring all of the pieces together, and in spite of the odds, create a perfect whole. How can we not stand in wonder when we witness this feat? Because when you understand all that can go wrong, you understand how delicate, dangerous and miraculous this balance is.

To think of one's ancestors, to send the mind back in time, far back to the multitude of women that make up one's family tree, women who lay on beds or on floors, or perhaps outside on the ground, and labored through a successful delivery without anesthesia or antibiotics, and lived, actually survived birth and, at least for her generation, continued the line of her ancestors, how can one not stand up and cheer when a birth is successful?

"We are the descendants of those who survived, those who succeeded in giving birth," Ellison writes. Perhaps if I, too, had not been witness to two different birth stories, the power of this truth would not stop me cold. Perhaps it would not have inspired me to call my mother and question her about the life of her grandmothers (each bore thirteen children and lived to be old women) and her great-grandmothers and any other woman's fate in our family history she could remember. Perhaps late at night it would not send my mind racing back in time to the ghosts of faceless women, some surviving birth, some not.

My first birth story is my own, dangerous, messy, and grim, its good outcome still a mystery to the medical world; and my second is Norah's, smooth and healthy, with only four pushes resulting in a perfect seven pound baby girl.

April Baby

A baby's presence exerts a consistent and persistent
domination over the outer and inner lives of every
member of a household. Because these members
must reorient themselves to accommodate his
presence, they must also grow as individuals and
as a group. It is true to say that babies control and
bring up their families as it is to say the converse. A
family can bring up a baby only by being brought
up by him. His growth consists of a series of
challenges to them to serve his newly developing
potentialities for social interaction.

Erik H. Erikson's, *Identity: Youth and Crisis*

"So what do you think of your baby sister?" My daughter
lies in bed, rubbing her tiny washcloth between her fingers, and
stares up at the ceiling.
"I like her," she says. "Do you like her?"
I nod. "I like her a lot."
We say nothing for a few minutes. I stare at my daughter's
face, at the red scar on her forehead, a straight line the size of a
matchstick; a reminder of just how little control I have. I look at
each moving part of her differently now: the eyes shift and focus,
the legs bend and jump and run, the throat swallows, the heart
beats, the kidneys cleanse, the brain functions as it should.
"Can the baby swim?" She asks.
"No, the baby can't swim yet."
"Can I teach her?" Her eyes widen at the very idea.
"When you learn to swim, then you can teach her." I say.

My daughter rolls over to face the wall. She is tired from the trip to Indianapolis, and happy to be back in her own bed. I do not move, I rub her back, listening to her breathe.

"Go do the dishes," she says.

She reaches her hand over and pats my arm, a gesture of benevolent indifference. I stand up and walk to the door. I understand now, more than before, how motherhood is a constant lesson in humility.

"Your daddy already did them," I say; an innocent lie out of loyalty to feminism and my duty to break stereotypes. But she is already asleep.

When Erikson explores the term identity crisis he writes, "it may be a good thing that the word 'crisis' no longer connotes impending catastrophe."

Yes, it is a good thing.

Last September when I found myself in the middle of a "crisis," there seemed to be no way out, no way to enact my long-favored strategy of willing it away. Looking back now it seems like fate that I should find myself sitting in a booth in McDonald's across from my sixteen-year-old brother who was also suffering from a crisis of his own; one that I soon realized was not so different than my own. 'Growing up' was the cause of his crisis, and it turned out to be the cause of mine as well. When I think back to the vacant expression on his face I understand that, in a way, he was in mourning, something had been lost amidst the physical and mental changes that had seized him one summer day, something had been irretrievably lost: his childhood, and all the comforts and safety that had gone along with it. To find oneself in a place unknown, but unable to go back and too afraid to move forward, what does one do? For a teenager, I suppose you lock yourself in your room, listen to really loud music, spend hours on the phone bitching to your friends about nothing of import, and just ride it out; until one day you wake up to find that you feel better, undeniably changed, but somehow stronger, finally ready to open the door again.

That night in September when I lay in bed reading the homemade baby food book, it was then that I realized that something had been lost, that my ability to carry another child had been taken away from me, and that I would never get it back. For me, an adult, a wife and a mother responsible for the well-being of a 3-year-old, hiding in my room and listening to really loud music all night long was not an option. So what followed was weeks and months of my own form of hiding: pretending, denying, acting; utilizing all the tricks I had learned in an attempt to wipe away the anger and sadness over this loss, and to run from the drama that I had deemed so invasive, so suffocating.

In many ways the darkness that came over me that night made no sense: I had found a loving woman to carry a child for me, and the embryo had taken hold, it was growing, and in nine months it would be born, despite me and my woes. The belief that I had already 'grown up,' that I had complete control over the course of my life and the lives of my children, and therefore needed no further help or guidance, this mistaken belief impeded my vision, distorted my understanding of what it means to love and to work, to rejoice and to be content, in essence to grow up. I missed important clues in the literal meaning of growing up: to mature, to change, to move, to adjust, to adapt. To accept that growth is essential to our minds and bodies if we wish, like John Adams, to continue living full and meaningful lives into old age, is also to accept the unpredictable nature of life as it unfolds. So much of what was mourned in my loss — of identity, of the physicality of childbirth — was embedded in the exchange between memories and the inevitability of growing up. These forces of life move in tandem, to deny or resist this truth is where the suffering lies. I mistook drama for the story line, drama is simply the spark, the ascendency of change that, whether deemed good or bad, opens up to the possibility of much more.

***

When I think about the first time I held my baby daughter, those few moments form in my mind in the present tense, as if it is happening in this instant. She stares up at me, she does not blink, her eyes open wide, their color dark, opaque as stone. I walk with her to the corner of the room and turn my back to the nurses and doctors, to my husband and Norah, and I look down at this child and with my eyes staring back into hers, I apologize.

I apologize for not being brave, for not standing up for her over the past nine months, as I should have. She deserves far more; I promise her more. She still stares up at me, her expression now one of exhaustion, and I lean close to her, pressing my face against the soft warmth of her skin, and I say, thank you.

Acknowledgements

I would like to thank my agent, Elizabeth Sheinkman, whose wisdom, guidance, and friendship is immeasurable. To Andy Zhang for reading this book as both an editor and a father. To John Palmer, Robert Pack, David Baine, and Susan Richards Shreve for their gifts of writing, teaching, and enduring encouragement.

I am forever grateful to Corinne Buckalew for taking this book under her wing, and for her friendship and unwavering support. To Amy Kimball, Kim Church, Sophia Volandes, Farah Roessner, Marybeth Dyson, Patti Dyson, Susan Smith Hendrickson, Michelle Schlesinger, George Hodgman, Graciela Meltzer, Sharon Lickerman, Sarah Outman Brophy, Frank Celenza, Jamie Junghans, Philip and Margret Delves Broughton, Nicole Webster, Marcea Driscoll, and Justin Palmer, for encouragement and advice. To Terri Edersheim, Sidney Wu, and Orli Etingin, words will never be enough. To Sara Switzer, for her friendship, brilliance, and escapes to Lowood.

To my mother and father for their support from the very beginning; my two brothers for keeping life interesting; to my grandfather, James, for a lifetime of valued advice; and to my late grandmothers for their legacies. To my mother and father-in-law, for providing the ultimate parenting example. Para Elsa Gagnay, mi amiga, mi hermana, y un regalo en mi vida. To Hilary Hanafin for the years she has dedicated to helping women. To Nancy Scudder, whose generosity and goodness will stay with me and my family for generations to come.

To my girls, you two are even better than the dream.

And finally to Patrick Dyson, the wondrous boy, who continues to inspire me.

Credits

Samuel Bercholz and Sherab Chodzin Kohn, Editors, *The Buddha and His Teachings* (Boston: Shambhala Publications, 1993), pp. 92, 93, 161, 165.

Sue Erikson Bloland, *In the Shadow of Fame: A Memoir by the Daughter of Erik H. Erikson* (New York: Penguin Group, 2005), pp. 50, 51, 52.

Andre Dubus, *Selected Stories* (New York: Vintage Books, 1996), pp. 20, 27, 39.

Peter T. Ellison, *On Fertile Ground: A Natural History of Human Reproduction* (Cambridge, Massachusetts: Harvard University Press, 2001), pp. 5, 7.

Erik H. Erikson, *Identity: Youth and Crisis* (New York: W.W. Norton & Company, Inc., 1968), pp. 92, 110, 113, 136, 139.

Lawrence J. Friedman, *Identity's Architect: A Biography of Erik H. Erikson* (Cambridge, Massachusetts: Harvard University Press, 1999), p. 19.

Elaine R. Gordon, *Mommy, Did I Grow In Your Tummy? Where Some Babies Come From* (Santa Monica, California: EM Greenberg Press, Inc., 1992), pp. 1, 2, 18, 19, 21, 25, 27.

Jerry Leiber and Billy Edd Wheeler, *Jackson*, 1963.

Betty Jean Lifton, *Journey of the Adopted Self* (New York: Basic Books, 1994), pp. 3, 4.

Connie Linardakis, *Homemade Baby Food Pure and Simple* (Roseville, California: Prima Publishing, 2001), pp. 68, 82, 186.

David McCullough, *John Adams* (New York: Simon & Schuster, 2001), pp. 568, 570, 571, 572, 590, 591.

Lorrie Moore, *Birds of America* (New York: Alfred A. Knopf, Inc., 1998), p. 253.

Adrienne Rich, *Of Woman Born: Motherhood As Experience and Institution* (New York: W.W. Norton & Company, 1986), p. 218.

Hans Sebald, *Adolescence: A Social Psychological Analysis* (Englewood Cliffs, New Jersey: Prentice-Hall, Inc., 1984), pp. 3, 4, 94.

Ayelet Waldman, "Truly, Madly, Guiltily" *The New York Times*, March 27, 2005.

Also by Aberdeen Bay

Falling

a memoir

At 18 years of age, Clint Pearson was a rock climber and local track star, and despite his long hair and carefree dress, he was maniacally driven. Even after being diagnosed with multiple sclerosis (MS), he continued to climb mountains and take risks, unmindful of the dangers. He shunned commitment and saw women as trophies, that is, until he met Ursula. A South African of East Indian descent, Ursula had grown up under the shroud of apartheid and had nurtured a healthy supply of caution in the process. At first she sought to maintain her distance from the brash and disheveled American, but after Clint and Ursula found themselves in a car, at night, inside a redwood forest, nuptials were soon to follow. Their differences were extreme but so too were their feelings for each other, and as Clint plodded through medical school, becoming emotionally entangled in the poignant dramas of his patients, the marriage remained strong. Then during residency training, financial pressures intensified, leisure time vanished, and Clint's MS progressed despite several medicines. On one occasion, MS medication even precipitated a high fever, and Clint's body had to be packed in ice. The marriage ultimately survived both Clint's declining health and his residency, but the MS continued to progress, making Clint's mountain-climbing ambitions increasingly unrealistic. Yet he remained an adventurer, a climber at heart. Would he push ahead only to stumble and fall or could Ursula and his patients somehow teach him to climb mountains of a different kind?

Author: Clint Pearson & Ursula Pearson
Publisher: Aberdeen Bay
ISBN-13: 978-1-60830-012-9
ISBN-10: 1-60830-012-9

Breinigsville, PA USA
26 August 2009
222979BV00001B/21/P